Husband-Coached Childbirth

By ROBERT A. BRADLEY, M.D.

1817

Harper & Row, Publishers

NEW YORK, EVANSTON, AND LONDON

LIBRARY OF CONGRESS CATALOG CARD NUMBER: 65-20994

This book is dedicated to those brave pioneers of change who dare to stand out as different in the crowd of conformity.

Contents

Foreword

Human beings usually give birth to one child at a time. And it takes nine lunar months from conception to the birth of a child. Hence, the preservation of the human species for the two million or so years that man has been on this earth has always been a near thing. It is therefore understandable that pregnancy and especially the birth of a child should have been invested with special value, as witnessed by the customs, ceremonials, rituals, and other practices with which these events are associated in all societies.

In every human society the birth of a child has been welcomed as the dramatic event it is, the unifying event that binds husband and wife and children together as no other event in the life of a family can. This was still the case even in the technologically advanced societies of the West in which, in the earlier part of this century, the child was usually born at home with a midwife assisting. In the warm and familiar ambience of the home the whole family could be involved in the birth of the child, and quite often it was the husband who assisted at the delivery, whether he was prepared to do so or not. But with the increasing shift to the hospital delivery room in which to have the baby—and 96 per cent of our women now have their babies in hospitals—the birth of a baby became mechanically routinized, and no longer a matter of family participation. Unfortunately, we—especially in the United States—have become increasingly mechanized, so that today we feel very strongly that if we can take anything out of human hands and especially out of the human heart and put it through a machine, we have made progress. Indeed, we flatter ourselves that we can make machines that think like human beings, while not always pausing to reflect that in the process we have also succeeded in making millions of human beings that can feel and think like machines. It is a sorry reflection.

A hospital is a splendid place, but it is not, in my view, a place in which the most beautiful celebration in the history of a family, the welcoming of a new member into it, should occur. That event should be celebrated where it belongs, in the bosom of the family, in the home. Dr. Bradley, in this admirable book does not quite agree. I am fully aware of the grounds of his disagreement, and I respect them, but on that point I believe this is no place to argue. I shall be producing a book on that subject in the future, and I shall be content to leave it to the future to arbitrate between us. But on virtually every other point I am in full agreement with Dr. Bradley, and I believe his book to be one of the most important contributions to the re-humanization of obstetrical practice that has been published in this century. If we can't yet have babies at home, the next best thing is to bring the home into the hospital. Something of this I attempted to do in proposing the idea of rooming-in more than twenty years ago.[1] Toward this end Dr. Bradley has made a monumentally important step in the right direction by bringing the father into the whole program of preparation for birth. It is not merely the revolutionary advance of having the father present during his wife's labor and the birth of their child in the "delivery room," but the sharing, insofar as that is possible for the male, of the pregnancy with his wife during the whole nine months thereof. Dr. Bradley is concerned to restore something of the ease and happiness, the security and the bountifulness as a human experience of pregnancy and birth to

[1] Ashley Montagu, "Some Factors in Family Cohesion. *Psychiatry*, vol. 7, 1944, pp. 349-352.

mother, father, and children. He requires no special understanding of technical problems—he explains them all with hardly ever resorting to a single one, in a breezy vernacular style that will endear him to all mothers and fathers. What Dr. Bradley *is* interested in is in making the birth of a baby an experience that mother and father can look forward to with pleasure, experience with joy, and make the foundation of an ever-firmer bond between them.

Dr. Bradley is an experienced and thoroughly reliable guide. He is a pioneer, and this is a pioneer book. The mothers and fathers who will read it will feel like pioneers, too, if, as I hope, they decide to adopt and follow Dr. Bradley's recommendations, for they will be pioneering in the most important of all frontiers: the making of good human beings in a good family. The family is the basis of society. As the family is, so is the society, and it is human beings who make a family—not the quantity of them, but the quality of them. As a contribution toward improving the quality of the family Dr. Bradley's book is of major importance. It brings that institution down from the abstract level of sociological discussion to the firm ground of what one does in order to make the meaning of a word achieve the action it produces. In other words, this is a beautifully practical book that potential parents can use as the compass by which to steer their way into the safe harbor of happily born children in a happy family where everyone is given the opportunity to inherit his birthright, which is development—without the obfuscating and damaging effects of an outmoded and wrongheeded traditional obstetrics.

—ASHLEY MONTAGU, PH.D.
Princeton, N.J.

Husband-Coached Childbirth

1

Introduction

THE ADMINISTRATOR of Porter Memorial Hospital in Denver, Colorado, called our office recently. He had received a request from the Canadian Broadcasting Corporation for permission to film a documentary on husband-coached natural childbirth for presentation on their program THIS HOUR HAS 7 DAYS.

Mrs. Merle Grosman, of Toronto, a natural childbirth mother herself and a member of the Natural Childbirth Association, had initiated the idea and had written to ask if we had patients who would cooperate.

In discussing it with her we decided to utilize a woman having her first baby. There is a misconception promoted by the unknowing that having a baby by natural childbirth might be possible after having had other babies but not with the first!

Accordingly we contacted our due or overdue primiparas (first pregnancies), and after Mr. Tom Kosh, director, and his crew of cameramen arrived, these wives were photographed with their husbands at class, doing prenatal exercises, etc., as participants in mental and physical preparation for childbirth. Then everyone waited patiently for one of them to go into labor.

The law of the perversity of nature in general and pregnant women in particular manifested itself in that we had had many births just before our Canadian visitors arrived, then had to wait a week before one went into labor. This served to illustrate again

1

that babies cannot read calendars and that doctors cannot tell when labor will begin.

As an honorary life member of the Toronto Natural Childbirth Association I was very much honored to be chosen to illustrate the great principles involved. I was also embarrassed that it took so long before a patient went into labor. I was bound by medical principles not to interfere with the development of a baby by forcing or inducing labor for anyone's convenience, so everyone waited.

Finally at midnight one night the phone rang and Mr. and Mrs. Gary Petersen announced they were on their way to the hospital. They were met at the hospital entrance by the somewhat sleepy but efficient TV camera crew of the CBC, who carefully followed the course of labor and birth with cameras and sound recorders. The visitors were intrigued and delighted by the calm self-assurance of these two young people who confidently went about the happy business of bearing a child as they had each been trained to do.

The husband had "signed in" for his wife while the nurse in attendance had performed the "prep." He then joined his wife, to remain with her throughout labor and birth and share the requested privilege of walking back with her from the "delivery" room.

Their gay, happy chatter as they strolled together in the early stages of labor would be rhythmically interrupted by uterine contractions. As her labor picked up in intensity they returned to the labor room and concentrated on their respective tasks. The old term "labor pains" just couldn't properly be applied here, for the observers could see no evidence of pain. The husband busily cranked the bed flat, arranged an extra pillow under his wife's raised knee as she turned on her side and assumed the "running" position of early first-stage labor which she had learned in class. During the contractions the young mother would calmly lie curled up, peacefully close her eyes, and automatically relax all the muscles of her body. The young husband tenderly placed a guiding hand on his wife's abdomen and directed her diaphragmatic breathing. He would also lean over and maintain a constant soft whispering in his wife's ear during this interval. The observing guests could not make out his words, but the endearing tone of his voice made apparent that the content was indeed the repetitious love "gobbledygook" with which she was so familiar. In prenatal classes the husbands are instructed to repeat verbally during contractions the intimate "love line" which was so effective in the moonlight originally and started the chain of events leading to the pregnancy.

When the muscle contractions of the uterus subsided, the chatter resumed, to be momentarily interrupted again rhythmically as the uterus went about its work uninhibited. Between contractions he would rhymically massage his wife's low back "saddle" area, accompanied by murmurs of approval from her. Whenever a contraction occurred the same calm pattern of relaxation, abdominal breathing, and love talk would be automatically repeated. As time went on the husband occasionally slipped ice chips in his wife's mouth with a spoon to counter the drying effect of mouth breathing, which is part of total relaxation during contractions. The couple performed their respective tasks calmly, automatically, with light chatter between contractions. The observers from Toronto were impressed by the obvious fact that here were two people working happily together. Each knew, without being told, exactly what they were about.

As time went on the interval between contractions gradually became shorter, the "chatter" accordingly gradually diminished, and the parents became more and more concentrated on their respective tasks. As each said, when asked later, they completely forgot about the presence of the observers; they were too busy.

The idea of some sort of medication being utilized in such an efficient peaceful performance never occurred to the performers and seemed ludicrous to the observers. The close relationship between husband and wife, the total dependence upon each other, was heart-warming to see—that it truly "takes *two* to tango" was never more manifest. Again the obvious ego-deflating question was put to me as the obstetrician: "Who needs a doctor for this?" My occasional vaginal examinations to determine the dilatation of the cervix constituted rather rude interruptions which momentarily disrupted the smooth working pattern of the process. They obviously got along better when the doctor wasn't around. I answered their question by stressing again that the doctor's role is vital in the preliminary preparation of two people, not in the performance. A swimming coach is necessary only during the learning period; after completion of the course we are mainly interested observers.

As labor progressed the parents became oblivious to anything or anyone as they carefully concentrated on the job at hand. This concentration was enhanced by the quiet, hushed "bedroom" atmosphere which is maintained in the labor rooms of this hospital. The importance of such an atmosphere is stressed as part of nurses' training in a course indoctrinating the principles of natural childbirth, which is part of the curriculum of the associated Union College Department of Nursing.

"Labor" is what the term implies, hard work, and although mothers are trained deliberately to relax all muscles during the uterine muscle's contractions, the uterus is of sufficient size and power as a muscular organ to produce perspiration in the mother in the later stages of labor. The husband's role included occasionally stepping out in the hall to cool a washcloth in cold water and apply it tenderly to the perspiring brow of his wife. Such seemingly trivial acts reduce the tasks of nurses and direct the gratitude of a mother to the one she loves, her husband.

Between contractions, at the wife's request, her position would be alternated occasionally by the husband's changing the bed to the contour chair, propped-up position and with his adjusting the two pillows to support his wife's arms. Again the familiar talk and cooperation would be evident.

The labor progressed to the transition stage, and the husband gently encouraged the deeper breathing techniques associated with this stage, knowing the need for change. The young mother shortly announced the urge to "push," ushering in the second stage of labor. After a short vaginal check by the doctor to verify the complete opening of the cervix, the pillows were adjusted by the husband behind his wife's shoulders and she was coached in assuming the squatting position in the elevated bed, the deep chest-breathing technique followed by long breath-holding, and the expulsive pushing with contractions. After a few pushes in bed the husband, doctor, and observers changed into "scrub suits," caps, and masks in the doctor's lounge while the attending nurses wheeled the mother to the nearby delivery room.

The husband took his place at the head of the delivery room table on the "daddy stool" which prior to natural childbirth was occupied by an anesthetist. He resumed his coaching of the breathing technique, adjusted the supporting pillows during each contraction to fit the contours of his wife's shoulders and back as she calmly held her breath, arched her back forward, and pulled her knees back under her armpits in the full squatting position on the downward tilted delivery table. This position served to open wide the soft tissues of the birth canal to allow gradual descent of the infant. Because of the degree of additional exertion required of the mother in this stage, ice chips are no longer allowed, and the husband utilized the cold moist washcloth not only to wipe away perspiration from her brow but to have his wife bite on between contractions to maintain moisture on her lips, as he had been trained to do.

In this, the second stage, the infant had passed from the uterus into the vaginal canal, and the uterus now slowed down in the frequency of contractions with longer intervals between. This resulted in a return of the chatter between wife and husband. The observers were again impressed by the calm, peaceful atti- tude of the parents as they conversed between contractions about whether the baby would be a girl or a boy, and eagerly looked forward to knowing soon. The husband made an admiring comment on his wife's ability to hold her breath during contractions.

As the baby was passed into the world, announcing her arrival with a lusty yell, the mutual exclamations of delight, "It's a girl!" by husband and wife, the shiny-eyed wonder at the miracle of this new life, the mutual pride in accomplishment manifested by husband and wife, made a picture of wholesome togetherness bordering on ecstasy.

After holding the baby low for a few minutes to allow blood in the placenta to siphon through the umbilical cord back into the baby, the doctor then handed the infant to the mother to hold. This first real meeting with her child is accompanied by such a delighted joyous expression on the mother's face that the husband, ready with his camera, recorded this important moment as a permanent record for the baby book.

With natural childbirth the total absence of anesthetics and anesthesia machines allows even flashbulb cameras to be safely used at this hospital.

While the parents were exuberantly examining the baby, I pointed out to the observers that with a few pushes before the actual birth I had performed the little cut (episiotomy) of the mother's flesh without any anesthetic and without objective evidence that she realized it had been done. Upon questioning her now, I found she had not known or felt it. God's anesthetic of properly applied pressure works magnificently for this purpose.

The umbilical cord was then clamped and cut while the mother was holding the baby. The baby was then put at the mother's side for the first introduction to breast feeding. The purpose of this was not primarily nourishment but to activate the breast-uterine reflex which stimulates uterine contractions to separate the placenta and decrease bleeding from the placental site. During this period of handling and nursing the child, husband and wife literally had their heads together. Their constant "parent talk" to the baby, calling it by name—Kirsten Lynn—and expression of delight to each other were accompanied by intimate expressions of mutual love, which made all the attendants feel like intruders. While the parents were playing with the baby I injected novocaine in the edges of the little cut (the first and only medication administered) and put in the necessary stitches—completely ignored by both parents. They were so absorbed in studying the baby, counting fingers and toes, commenting on whose hair color it inherited, etc., that they paid no attention.

The mission accomplished, each parent was then given a complimentary glass of iced orange juice—for the mother to replenish blood sugar, depleted from its utilization by the uterus, and to correct the drying effect of mouth breathing during labor; for the father as a token of appreciation for his important participation and to maintain the great principle of sharing this beautiful experience with his wife.

The mother then expressed the desire to walk back from the delivery room. She was given her robe and slippers, and with the baby in one arm, a glass of orange juice in the other hand, and a beaming, proud husband alongside, she strolled happily out the door and down the hall—mission accomplished. A helpful nurse, using the husband's camera, took a final picture of this new family group.

In the last sixteen years as a teacher of natural childbirth I have seen this happy series of events repeated thousands of times. To our visitors from Toronto it was a new and never to be forgotten experience. I was delighted to have our busy office hours interrupted a few hours later by the director and photographers stopping by to express their admiration and praise over the method, and their gratitude for the privilege of witnessing the birth. Most significant to me was that they had sent flowers to the new mother and were passing cigars around as enthusiastically as if each were the father of the baby! The spirit of joy and pride in accomplishment of a natural birth is indeed contagious.

2

The Theory of Natural Childbirth

To ANYONE like myself who grew up in God's great outdoors and witnessed the birth process in animals, other than human, the inevitable question is bound to arise: Why do all other animals peacefully and joyfully give birth unassisted? Why can't the human animal do this? What makes the difference?

Throughout my childhood I was fortunate enough to live on the outskirts of a small town in what amounted to a farming environment. We had a large barn that in the course of years was occupied by many domestic animals. We averaged from eight to ten cats, had horses, cows, goats, and a succession of dogs. In addition to these domestic animals the open countryside adjacent to our place afforded the opportunity to observe many wild animals. The birth processes I witnessed in these many creatures were attended with no objective evidence of pain or suffering. The opposite was true. The animal mother's eyes were radiant with joy and happiness.

This was brought back to my awareness not long ago. A sheep rancher, female variety, from a neighboring state had heard that I was a natural childbirth doctor, so she came to see me when she discovered her pregnancy.

I'll never forget her first visit. She was over six feet tall, dressed in the clothing of her trade—boots, levis, and Stetson hat. She stormed into the office with great strides, and loudly and firmly announced to our office girl and all present in the reception room that her husband had gotten her pregnant during the lambing season and "I just decided then and there if those dumb sheep can give birth to their young that easily, so can I. I'm just as smart as they are!" Let me assure you that after completion of our training course she was every bit as good as her word—she was indeed as smart as her sheep and a marvelous natural childbirth mother.

What, then, is the difference between human and other animals?

Are their bodies made differently? As a matter of fact they are remarkably similar. Cat and dog bodies are used in premedical anatomy studies due to the similarity of structures with identical name and function. Is it that they just can't experience pain? Following a natural childbirth newspaper article, an indignant letter to the editor asserted cats can have kittens without pain because they cannot feel pain as human beings do. I've often wondered if that misguided lady had ever stepped on a cat's tail in a darkened room, or rocked on a cat's paw with a rocking chair?

No, that's not an adequate explanation, for animals otherwise manifest pain when hurt.

What is the difference, then? Dr. Grantly Dick-Read proposed a theory to explain this difference as far back as 1932. No one paid much attention. In 1947 my wife happened to read his book *Childbirth Without Fear: The Principles and Practice of Natural Childbirth.* I had just started my postgraduate training in obstetrics. My M.D. degree was new and shiny, which meant I knew just about everything. How time and maturity can change that conception! At my aloofness she commanded, "Read it, you big lummox, it makes sense!" I hadn't been a doctor very long but I had been married eight years: I read it. It did make sense. It brought back to mind those puzzling questions that had been lingering since the days on the farm. Why the difference?

Dr. Dick-Read's theory was essentially that all other animals instinctively *do something* that keeps the birth process from hurting. They have built in know-how, called instinctual knowledge, and automatically do the right thing at the right time. Humans, apparently lacking this instinctual knowledge, do the wrong thing; and the wrong thing hurts and prolongs labor.

My mind mulled over this thing called animal instinct. What is it? No one knows, but there it is, and there it acts. Not only in labor and birth but also in swimming, or knowing what to do in water. Human beings are the only animals I could think of who drown when dropped in deep water; all other animals I could think of or could remember from my youth know how to swim, and do so immediately and perfectly when immersed. Also human animals are the only ones I know who need to take compasses along on hunting trips—so they can find their way back home! All other animals have "homing instinct"—you can't lose that cat even if you try! It will frequently get home before you.

Does that mean that we should curse our Creator because He apparently shortchanged us and "forgot" to give us this knowledge? No, we are really the superior animals, judging by the fact that when we visit the zoo we are on the outside of the cages and they are on the inside. God gave us a magnificent brain capable of abstract thinking, a high level of communicative ability, learning, retention, reasoning, etc. The current theory of natural childbirth is that we should study the animals and by intelligent reasoning learn to do through training and practice what they do by instinct. Or, to make a blunt comparison, a woman who doesn't know how to swim is given nine months' notice that she will be thrown in deep water. Let's assume that during that nine-month period she does not avail herself of classes where swimming is taught. This is as unreasoning as one who knows she is pregnant, does not know how to act in labor, and then during her nine months does not bother to attend classes in the conduct of labor. The results in both cases would be horrible to behold, particularly by someone who loves the participant.

Natural childbirth training displaces ignorance, superstition, fear, anxiety, and the resultant bodily tensions which are such obstacles in labor and in swimming. There is nothing more pleasurable to observe than an expert human swimmer frolicking in deep water. Similarly there is nothing more marvelous to behold than an expert, educated, trained human mother giving birth.

Dr. Dick-Read's principles disturbed me. Is it really necessary for women to suffer so in labor? Do they really have to be *delivered?* Must they lose all human dignity and self-control in labor from the drunken effect of medication given in the vain attempt to make labor pain-free? Does medication really make labor pain-free? If the answer to the latter question is not perfectly clear in your mind, I beg you, ask women who have tried the medication method! This brings to mind an article I read years ago written by an intelligent career woman, a journalist, as I recall. She had married late in life after a brilliant career, deciding in the last few months of fertility that she wanted to become a mother before nature shut off this function. Being a strong-willed person, she acted upon her decision and became pregnant. Being also a scientifically oriented person, she enthusiastically investigated the next logical question: "What's it like, having a baby? What am I to expect?" She found there were in existence two fundamental ways: One involved medication and anesthetics to relieve pain and being passively "delivered" of her baby. The other was the method of natural childbirth whose enthusiastic advocates disdained the "knock 'em out, drag 'em out" approach and actively gave birth to babies without any "pain relief" medication at all. She applied, sensibly, the old car slogan "Ask the man who owns one." She proceeded carefully to interview a group of mothers who had used the medicated method—"Between us girls, what was it really like to have a baby?" The answers were horrifying: "Never again!" "Worse pain I have ever known!" "Most terrible experience of my life!" She then interviewed natural childbirth mothers, and I heartily encourage any honest skeptic to do likewise. "It was wonderful!"—"Most beautiful experience of my life!" "How would anyone want to be asleep at such a wonderful moment?" Some of the mothers used Helen Wessel's new term "birth climax,"[1] subjectively comparing the feeling of birth with the emotional climax in love-making. Mrs. Wessel had three babies by medication, then three by natural childbirth. Experience is still the best teacher.

After seventeen years and well over seven thousand attended births by natural childbirth I have often stated that the only handicap I have found in the method is the super-enthusiasm of the parents afterward. They will talk your arm off. They are forever writing articles, e.g., Gina Lollobrigida, Julie Harris, Jan Sterling, Princess Grace of Monaco, one of the Dionne quintu-plets, and others. This very book is being written at the persistent insistence of my patients.

Back to the bewildered young doctor being nagged by a de-termined little wife. Dr. Grantly Dick-Read's approach sounded too simple, even oversimplified. But it might be true; maybe humans could imitate animals in labor and enjoy similar unmedi-cated births. But what is the scientific explanation? What is the mechanical and physiological action? I didn't know then, I don't know now, seventeen years later. I doubt if I'll ever know the academic explanation of why or how it works. However, being a clinician (one who does), I tried it out in 1947. I applied these principles and believe me, they *do* work. Women can give birth by the action of their own bodies. Women can enjoy the process of birth and add to their dignity by being educated to follow the example set by instinctive animals. Women can take joy and pleasure and bless God for the privilege of being women and being able to give birth, instead of showing snarling hostility toward the men who love them—because men don't have to have children.

[1] Helen Wessel, *Natural Childbirth and the Christian Family*, Harper & Row, Inc., 1963.

3
Where Do Husbands Fit In?

W<small>HAT DO MEN</small>—husbands, fathers—have to do with this? It's rather obvious that these "rats" start the whole business of pregnancy. Is that all they have to do?

Frankly back in 1947 when I timidly tried out the method, I never gave the fathers a second thought. This was not actually purposeful on my part but was very necessary, as my first experimental patients were out of wedlock, pregnant girls in a confinement home. I was assigned this home as part of my obstetrical training at the university. Because it was distant from the main campus and my chief put me in complete charge I decided to apply these principles of training and preparation and see for myself what the results would be.

The patients took to the classes like ducks to water. This was possibly related to the fact that by far the majority of them were above average intelligence (and some quite brilliant academically) and also they were quite bored. Their confinement began when their pregnant abdomen began to show, and although the administrators of the home did a fine job, the hours would drag. They welcomed with eagerness the chance to learn more about themselves and the labor to come. Careful indoctrination was carried out, teaching the subjective feelings of labor, explanations of anatomy, stages of labor, etc. They were then taught the objective actions of animals in these stages of labor and how they

13

should carefully imitate them when their turn came. (For details of conduct of labor see subsequent chapters.) To make the story more brief, they never missed any classes; they were ideal and cooperative in labor. Even though they would not be able to keep their babies, they obviously enjoyed having them. I even brought my wife over to observe the results of her persistence in getting me to try the method. The idea of "taking medicine" as part of labor and birth did not occur to these healthy young women. When we did episiotomies (small cuts), they were done without medication or anesthesia and without the patient being aware of the cuts. The simple injection of novocaine in the borders of the incision was used just prior to placing the few stitches—*after* passage of both the baby and placenta.

Being young, and therefore naïve, I enthusiastically proposed a planned control study in the main clinic at the university. I was thoroughly squelched by my superiors and laughed at by my colleagues. All well and good for O.W.'s (out of wedlocks), who are noted for cooperating so well with their doctors. Just don't try it on married women with a husband to put on a show of martyrdom for. It wouldn't work!

Husbands! I hadn't thought about them—mainly because there weren't any. I started thinking and fretting. Why should a woman, if she loved her husband and he loved her, put on a show of uncooperative martyrdom? Why were O.W.'s so much better patients, by medical reputation, than married women? It didn't make sense. I reasoned that the O.W.'s had a more cooperative interpersonal relationship with the doctors for the simple unflattering reason they didn't have anyone else to whom to relate. However, if they were married and had an ever-loving husband, that doctor would be a relatively unimportant figure. But what if they truly loved their husbands, who when their reassuring presence was needed weren't there? Then they would have to accept that poor substitute who *was* there, the doctor.

My head was in a whirl. Did just being a married woman make a woman a poor obstetrical patient? Again it didn't make sense.

Being a clinician by intent, I decided the only way to find out was to try it and see.

Accordingly I asked for volunteers in natural childbirth experiments from the world's second most impossible obstetrical patients—married pregnant nurses. The world's most impossible would be married pregnant female doctors.

The latter category are rare birds; there weren't enough available, although I succeeded in finding a few.

In the former category I was swamped with volunteers. Before I leave the wrong impression on the reader, the reason medically trained personnel are emotionally poor-risk patients (R.N.'s and M.D.'s) is simply that they know too much. They have seen and heard medicated maniacs in labor. They have witnessed forceps-bruised babies. Everything of a negative nature has been seared indelibly on their subconscious minds, to come back and haunt them later when they are pregnant.

As a teacher and dispeller of fear and anxiety I get no particular sense of personal accomplishment in preparing a country girl for the birth of her baby, a girl (like the sheep rancher) whose only association with the birth process has been the peaceful, joyful births of animals she has witnessed on the farm. There really isn't much for the doctor to do. But give me a woman whose soul has been seared with negativity, and when she gives birth, after our preparatory course, with joy and peace and without even associating medication with the act, then I feel a sense of accomplishment.

Accordingly I took the volunteer married R.N.'s. Why did they volunteer? I think an article written in the local paper by an R.N. mother gives the reason in the very title: "Better Start for Babies." Here were mothers who not only loved their husbands, but also loved their babies. "Please, Doctor, teach me how to have a pink baby that cries right away." They had observed, as assistants, the difference in the color, muscle tone, and immediate cry of a lusty, healthy, natural childbirth, unmedicated baby compared with the "Does your mother know you're out" label

sarcastically applied by nursery personnel to medicated anesthe-
tized mother's limp blue babies. The difference is obvious.

So I trained and indoctrinated the married nurses—however,
still ignoring husbands. Results? In spite of the "handicap" of
being married and being nurses, they were even more cooperative
than the O.W.'s. They were magnificent mothers. At this stage
of my medical career no husband, to my knowledge, had ever
been allowed in that forbidding no man's land known as delivery
room, where the great white father of authority, the doctor,
reigns supreme. I myself had accepted these traditions without
questioning. However an event happened to jar me out of my
intellectual conformity.

With these experimental mothers at that time, I had allowed
the husband in the labor room and frankly ignored him. When
it was time to go to no man's land he was automatically sent to
the waiting room for fathers as was customary. Looking back
now, I don't see how I could have been so callous about a fellow
man's feelings. At the time I was concentrating on a set pattern of
testing the different aspects of the theory. I sat by the side of
every experimental patient throughout the entire course of labor.
I deliberately mistreated those wonderful mothers at regular intervals by carefully studying them objectively when they performed as instructed, then for experimental purposes, coached
them to do the opposite of what I had observed animals doing. I
would then take notes on their objective appearance of pain, and
correlate it later with a questionnaire to get their subjective eval-
uation. I was the coach and in constant attendance. The husband
sat in the labor room and did nothing and said nothing. I began to
awaken to his importance when I noticed how much more calm
and cooperative the patient was when her husband was present. If
he left the room, even temporarily, the mother became anxious
and tense and relaxed poorly with contractions. It had not
dawned on me as yet to capitalize on this effect and turn the
coaching over to him. That came later.

The husband was still thoughtlessly dismissed to the waiting room when birth became imminent. His wife was taken to the delivery room for the medical convenience of gadgets: special bed, lights, etc. Such paraphernalia is designed for the convenience of the attendants only—the mother could readily give birth in the labor room bed, and some speed-ball mothers inadvertently demonstrated this with simple dexterity.

In those days, any time an experimental natural childbirth trained mother was in labor the word spread around the hospital with lightning speed. As this was a teaching hospital—both student nurses and medical students—there soon came to be quite a gathering of visitors: nurses, scrub ladies, students, interns, and residents (this is in order of their importance!).

One of these nurse volunteer patients was a very attractive girl. I had sat beside her and coached her throughout labor, and when the baby was born I slipped off my "sterile" gloves and leaned over the table to shake her hand formally and congratulate her on her performance and thank her for her cooperation as was my custom.

As I leaned over to grasp her hand, in her exuberant gratitude she suddenly grabbed me with both arms and kissed me soundly, exclaiming happily, "Oh, thank you, thank you for showing me how." My shoes were wet from the salt water that so liberally accompanies the baby's arrival and I lost my balance and fell awkwardly against my patient, to the hilarious amusement of the onlookers. It was soon the talk of the hospital and the source of many good-natured jibes about my "bedside manner" with attractive patients.

Kidding I had grown used to, but I was suddenly shocked to serious thought as I walked back from this joyful scene to the waiting room and saw the frightened, anxious, distraught face of the man whose love and affection had been shared with this woman to produce this child.

It struck me like a sledge hammer. What on earth was this lovely woman kissing *me* for? Why was I the object of her gratitude as a labor coach while her young lover sat uselessly in the waiting room, fearful and anxious over his sweetheart's safety, eagerly wishing to see the outcome of his love for her, the baby, yet deprived by isolation from the most meaningful emotional experience of their lives together?

The more I thought about it, the more ridiculous it seemed. The old adage that all pregnant women fall in love with their obstetricians came to my mind; of course they may, since their lovers are not allowed to be there to share with their wives this rich emotional experience of their lives together. Why shouldn't husbands be there? Why couldn't the role of labor coach, which as I had performed it this night had created such exuberant gratitude in the mind and soul of this mother, be performed by her husband? Was my ego in such a sad plight that it had to be constantly bolstered by pushing aside a real lover and accepting substitute favors from my patients? I felt more embarrassed the more I thought about it. I have been married now for twenty-five years to that same little nagging (God bless her) wife who insisted after reading Dr. Dick-Read's book that natural childbirth made sense. I am not the least bit interested in having my patients falling in love with me, but I feel deeply the responsibility, as an obstetrician, to see that the act of bearing a child makes them fall *more* in love with their husbands.

I did not dream then that such a simple logical decision could result in such a barrage of obstacles and opposition from many sides and for many years to come.

The opposition has never originated from the many mothers or their husbands, because once they were instructed in their role they were eager and looked forward to the birth. No, the opposition came from fellow doctors, administrators, and nursing supervisors—a rather formidable array.

Doctors oriented in the principles of natural childbirth presented no opposition, quite the contrary. However such doctors were then, and in most areas still are, in the minority. For such a radical innovation as husbands in delivery rooms we could not rely on a majority vote of the medical staff—then or now.

The hope for cooperative hospital rules lay in the acceptance of the administrator and his staff. Being in training at a university hospital where research was encouraged, I presented a program to the administrator as the trial of a new concept in obstetrics—total or psychosomatic obstetrics—adding psychological, emotional, and spiritual overtones as compared to the mechanical and purely medical aspects of childbearing.

After reassuring him of insurance coverage of husbands, pointing out that husbands represented not an additional person present but a substitute for the anesthetist, after promising to supply the new labor coach with suit, cap, and mask similar to those worn by doctors, permission for the trial was granted. That was many, many husbands-in-delivery-rooms ago. The fears of the unknowing objectors have proved groundless. No husband has fainted in the delivery room or otherwise made a nuisance of himself. On the contrary, he has added an element of humor and joy and has become very much a member of the team. And regardless of the opposition, he is on the team to stay. Acceptance of these new concepts is slow but sure. Max Planck has said, "A new scientific truth does not triumph by convincing its opponents and making them see the light, but rather because its opponents eventually die, and a new generation grows up that is familiar with it."

One member of this new generation, John Quinn, a student at Humboldt State College in Arcata, California, made newspaper headlines when he chained himself to his laboring wife in order to foil the hospital ban on his presence. His explanation (after police were summoned) is a classical example of the increased awareness of the younger generation: "I love my wife. I feel it's my moral right as a husband and father to be there." This basic human right—to share childbirth with your wife—is expressed in the lyrics of the song "The Green Leaves of Summer"—*It was so good to be young then, to be close to the earth and to stand by your wife at the moment of birth.*

Other young men have brought legal action against hospital

bans in order to achieve the same purpose. Chains and injunctions are things of the past now as hospital administrations are yielding to the demands of these young people to be able to share this important event in their lives.

Let us not lose sight of the great underlying principle that is fundamental to the concept of a husband as a participant in the birth process—preparation and training of both parents to achieve *birth* without the use of anesthetics rather than with the older medicated *delivery*. I have often said I would hesitate to bring a yellow cur dog into a delivery room to witness a medicated mother being put to sleep and her many times more sleepy baby being "delivered"; the dog would get sick! This concept was well illustrated by the French movie *The Case of Dr. Laurent*, which opened on a scene in a tiny village with a man leading a horse out of his stable and taking the horse down the street to other quarters. A bystander asked the man why he was taking the horse away. His answer was that the horse had become ill from the day-and-night screaming of a woman in labor in the nearby house. The movie went on to show the elderly doctor administering another hypo to the distraught woman.

Older hospital rules separating husband and wife in labor were meaningful and purposeful when established. This was in the era of what I have heard young natural childbirth enthusiasts disdainfully refer to as the "knock 'em out—drag 'em out" days. These rules were reasonable then, and husbands had no business being near their wives. However, in view of the increasing number of childbirth education programs stressing the importance of active participation in labor by both the husband and wife with the mutual goal of spontaneous birth, these husband-banning rules are obsolete.

Husbands have no business being with their wives in labor unless: (1) the wife has been trained how to perform in labor and has physically prepared her birth-giving muscles; (2) the husband has been prepared so that he understands how, why, and what his wife is doing, enabling him to coach, guide, and encourage her in her ennobling work. He should be well acquainted in advance with her appearance in the various stages of labor. By being prepared for her objective appearance he not only feels serene and self-confident through familiarity, but can apply his knowledge by acting as a coach to actually see to it that she performs properly. She, in turn, feels secure knowing that her ever-present coach not only loves her but knows what she is about and how to guide her. As one experienced natural childbirth mother peacefully expressed it, "As long as he's there I know he won't let me goof."

4

Preparation and First-Stage Labor

First-Stage Labor: What Do Animals Do?

ANIMAL FATHERS' presence in labor is unnecessary, as the animal mother can rely on her instinctive know-how and needs no coaching. However, your wife, lacking this instinct, must be guided, directed, and encouraged.

If your wife is to handle herself in labor as other animals do, let us carefully observe their conduct to see what we can learn. Although almost any species of lower animals would serve as an example, let's take one that is domesticated, say the cat or dog, for convenience, and observe them in labor.

The first observation will be that animals do not like to be observed in labor—by anyone. They become secretive, coy, and cunningly try to make this a private party. The family cat does not perform this deed out on the sidewalk or in any obvious place. It will, if left alone, probably perform at night and retire to the same location where it sleeps. It does not want distractions. There seems to be a great need to concentrate on the job at hand and the animal knows this need and resents distractions. Even a favorite dog, known for its good temper and loving nature, will snap or bite its master if disturbed in labor.

We have already gained a point in the necessity for training husbands as labor attendants. They must not do anything that will distract or disturb their wives during labor or the husband may be verbally snapped at. This does not mean the laboring mother (be it dog or human) has lost her love for the master or husband. Rather it points out the fundamental commandment of nature: Laboring mothers should not be disturbed or distracted; there is a great need for deep concentration by the mother. If this concentration is disturbed, pain and prolongation of labor result.

At a district convention of the I.C.E.A. (International Childbirth Education Association) held in Madison, Wisconsin, we were privileged to take a tour through the primate laboratories where Dr. Harry F. Harlow and his associates were studying mother-child relationships in rhesus monkeys. Their work involved the study of the results of early separation of baby monkeys from their mothers at an average of seven hours from birth and subsequent exposure of the babies to surrogate or substitute mothers of varying characteristics. I questioned the guide who was conducting the tour as to why they didn't separate the babies *immediately* after their birth. The answer was that, for purposes of the study, this would be ideal but that it was impossible. The mothers always gave birth at night, but when humans stayed up to separate the infant monkeys immediately, the mother's labor would become irregular and even cease because of the emotional disturbance created by the presence of the human intruder. If disturbing a mother's emotions in labor so drastically affected uterine action in rhesus monkeys, could this be true also in human mothers?

In lecturing student nurses it is stressed that the labor room should be darkened by pulling the shades in daylight. Although human mothers have apparently lost the instinctual ability to bear their young always at night, a darkened room is still of benefit. Labor rooms at night should be dimly illuminated from the sides, never by overhead lights—except momentarily during nurse or doctor examinations.

Now, back to the family cat or dog in labor. By quietly, even sneakily, approaching we observe additional factors involved.

1. *The need for darkness and solitude.* Bright lights are indeed disturbing. My attempts to take photographs of dogs and cats have been foiled by the indignant laboring mothers retreating to dark secluded places—usually physically out of reach of annoying humans—such as far under the house or barn.

2. *The need for quiet becomes obvious.* Any loud or unexpected noise disturbs the mother. Again we make the fervent plea to attendants in hospital labor sections to keep raucous noises down to a minimum. One careless, loud-mouthed, clanging nurse can undo hours of prenatal preparation and set the stage for another series of "Cruelty in Maternity Wards" articles,[1] justified examples of human mothers snapping at their disturbers in labor.

3. *The need for physical comfort* during first-stage labor is made manifest by animals in many ways. On the farm we could predict the imminence of labor when the pregnant cat would be seen carefully digging out a hollow place for its body in the warm earth under the barn. It would test out the area by lying in it, then diligently paw away any lump or irregular area until its body fit the cavity in the earth without any disturbing localized pressure. A few years ago our beloved family dog, a French poodle, was pregnant and the children noticed with delight how several days before the birth occurred the dog dutifully raided the soiled clothes basket in the basement, selecting articles of soft material, and laboriously dragged them up the steps to her basket in the kitchen. Here she meticulously lined the basket with them, turning around and carefully pawing away any lumps until she was satisfied with the comfortable contour. Wise mother that she was, she was upset by the attention her acts were bringing from the overly interested children and after the household was asleep, cunningly transferred her nest padding to a closet left open in the

[1] *Ladies Home Journal,* December 1958.

bathroom. She gave birth to her puppies peacefully and quietly during the night without arousing a soul—much to the disappointment of the children.

Observation of animals, then, points out the need for a comfortable position of the mother's body during labor. For years human mothers—and their doctors!—have been guessing wrong when labor will begin. How does the animal mother having her first pregnancy know in advance to so prepare? I'll leave the answer to that "how" question to the academic doctors—I can't answer it and, as yet, neither can they—but as a clinical doctor may I strongly point out that animals *do know* and that this observed fact is not weakened in the least by our human ignorance of *how* they know. The scientific eye of human learning is just now beginning to look timidly into the function of animal brains and instinctive abilities—and it has a long way to go.

4. *The need for physical relaxation.* These itemized needs are not mutually exclusive. Relaxation even in animals takes concentration. When this concentration is disrupted (by bright lights, loud noises, uncomfortable positions, presence of strangers) the animal tenses up, and tensing up during uterine contractions produces in animals the same thing it does in human mothers in first-stage labor-pain! Again we academically do not know *how*, but we jolly well know clinically that it *does*.

We encourage any human mother not to "believe" a word we state on the concepts we are teaching. We respect intelligent, honest skepticism. Being a man, and therefore destined never to know the actual feelings of labor, I have always, from the first experimental patient years ago to the current one in labor, challenged them to "believe" nothing but to "try" everything proposed, and then tell me if there is a difference. I throw this challenge to the reader: Carefully coach your wife in first-stage labor in the details of relaxation, then ask her to tense her voluntary muscles deliberately (any muscle—it doesn't matter which) during the next uterine contraction and then tell you the effect of such deliberate tensing. Try it and see what she says! No wonder the animal mother will try her best to avoid such disturbances and actually attack even a loved human being if he persists in disturbing her concentration!

Animal mothers are observed to lie absolutely still and physically relaxed during the contraction of their uterine muscles. Like efficient athletes, the muscles not being utilized in the event are completely inactive and relaxed, enabling the energies of the body to be more effectively directed to the one that is being utilized. My long-suffering wife has laughingly said that I bore friends to death by seeing manifestations of natural childbirth principles in everything and anything. The basketball player going in for a set-up shot at the basket is graceful and lithe—the arm not being used in this one-arm shot is limp and relaxed. The football player getting set to kick the crucial place-kick that may win the game is a picture of deliberate relaxation as he shakes tension from his shoulders and arms to increase the effectiveness of his leg muscles. The mother, whether by instinct or training, who deliberately loosens her other muscles during her uterine muscles' contraction is rewarded by comfort (nature's reward for helping rather than hindering birth) and by effectively producing the desired result (shortening of time required).

5. *The need for controlled breathing.* Animals breathe in first-stage labor in the same fashion as in sleep. Because labor is what the term implies—hard work—the breathing is deeper and, as labor progresses, more rapid. Here confusion arises as some species of animals do not perspire. Body heat is increased due to the forcefulness of the uterine contractions. In animals with perspiration mechanisms, and this includes the human, cooling is achieved by perspiration. Other animals are observed to break into panting type of breathing, at intervals, which serves as their particular mechanism to cool their body. Most animals, particularly if the environment is warm, breathe through open mouths rather than the narrower air passages of the nostrils. This may be related to the need for a greater volume of air or, as some have

suggested, the relaxation of the jaw muscles as part of the over-all state of generalized relaxation.

6. *The need for closed eyes and the appearance of sleep.* Again this is probably only a manifestation of the need for absolute and total concentration. It results in the label of the first stage of labor as that of the "sleep" stage. Animals return to their sleep place, lie, breathe, and look as if they were asleep during first-stage labor. The irritation that they manifest at the presence of humans may be related to their distrust and need for keeping an eye on the intruder even when the human is inactive. This again interferes with the increased ability to concentrate that comes from shutting out visual stimuli. Closed-eye concentration seems to be a necessary aspect of their job.

What Should Human Mothers Do?

The answer to this question by the hypothesis of the natural childbirth concept is, of course, that human mothers should do the same thing!

Because of slight structural differences of the human body, and because of considerable differences in the human soul, we now need to take the animal observations we have made and apply them one by one to this complex and highly developed mixed-up animal known as the human being. What works for other animals may work for us. Let's try it.

Animals like quiet, dark, comfortable secluded places to give birth to their young. They do not like the presence of strangers. Well, we have a big problem right off the bat. Doctors want human mothers to have babies in hospitals, and these requirements would hardly be achieved by the environment of *any* hospital. They are most nearly met by the environment of a mother's bedroom in her own home and the reassuring nearness of familiar and loved faces rather than those of strangers.

As a doctor and advocate of natural childbirth I can have no arguments with Ashley Montagu and other authorities on human relations who contend that from a bacteriological, sociological, psychological, moral, and spiritual standpoint human babies should be born at home. The home environment appears to best fulfill the requirements I have itemized. However, as an obstetrician I must in all honesty insist that babies shall or should be born in hospitals. Deuced nuisance that hospitals are to all concerned, my medical conviction takes precedence. Why? Because there is an irreducible incidence of complications in human obstetrics, and hospitals are best equipped for immediate management and correction of these complications. Some complications can be foretold in advance, but others cannot. It would be convenient to have the many uncomplicated births at home and only the complicated ones at the hospital, but this simply cannot be, as we doctors cannot guarantee in advance which is which. Some compassionate doctors oriented on the principles of family-centered childbirth are compromising their medical judgment and catering to the wishes of their patients for the peaceful seclusion of their own homes and the earnestly desired presence of their husbands at the birth of their babies. I wholeheartedly disagree. We must not alter the great advances already made in the medical and mechanical aspect of obstetrical management.

Natural childbirth principles should add to, not detract from, the established principles of obstetrics. They should add what has been lacking, proper and complete preparation of the mind and soul of both husband and wife for their introduction into parenthood. In our series about 3 per cent of our patients need Caesarean sections. Of the remainder who can have their babies through the vaginal route, 96.4 per cent achieve spontaneous, uncomplicated, unanesthetized births that could have been properly managed at home. However, there is still that 3.6 per cent who need hospital-equipped management of unforeseeable complications.

From a medical standpoint, then, babies should be born in the hospital. This does not, however, alter one bit the importance of the great principles we follow. It does present the formidable task of altering the hospital environment to make it conform with the home environment as closely as possible.

Years ago when the full realization of this task became apparent, it was almost overwhelming. Maternity hospitals were cold, gaunt, impersonal halls of barren stone cluttered with strange gleaming steel gadgets of awesome appearance, ruled over and run by eagle-eyed matrons policing a list of rules and regulations that would choke a horse. About as remote from a secluded home environment as one could get. Guilt-ridden husbands were glared at and told to stay in the waiting room—that chamber of horrors where nervous, distraught, useless, cigarette-smoking clowns paced the floor. Could such an introduction to fatherhood be related to the current lowered status of manhood and the rising incidence of divorce?

The need for change was as obvious as the task was formidable. A few "Daniels" who dared to be different dug in to effect a change. The home environment must be reproduced as much as possible in the hospital. Many little changes—in decor, subdued noise, more humane, and warmer attitudes by personnel—were brought about. However, the most important factor, and the one most desired by the mothers, was the inclusion of the husband with the wife throughout labor and birth. Yet in most localities it is only recently that this has been achieved.

Today through the noble efforts of many devoted workers family-centered childbirth, which includes having husbands in delivery rooms, is being introduced into more and more hospitals.

Having selected a hospital and a doctor that encourage you to share childbirth with your wife, let's get back to how you are going to help your wife imitate the lower animals in the conduct of her labor. Most family-centered maternity hospitals have a preliminary guided tour for you and your wife. By all means take advantage of this tour and become familiar with the appearance of the labor and birth room. Knowing where you're going and what it looks like is important too.

There are certain necessary nuisances you must take in stride when you enter the hospital with your wife in labor. She will be separated from you temporarily to have her "prep" and enema. She does not need your guidance for these little preliminaries and you will be busy signing in for her at the admissions desk. Part of being a good husband is being a good provider, so for heaven's sake contact the business office of the hospital in advance during her pregnancy and have clearly in mind what is required of you at the time of admission. This varies with each hospital and should have been worked out in advance. While you are attending to this, the nurse on duty will have shaved your wife's perineal area (surrounding the vagina) and administered the cleansing enema. The rectum is adjacent to the birth canal and when emptied makes more space available for the baby. (See Chapter 5.)

You will now be escorted to your wife in the labor room. Some hospitals require you to remove outside clothing and don a father's "hatching jacket," as our husbands fondly call these coats. Wear it with pride. It is the label of a birth coach and is indeed a mark of distinction.

Living in colorful Colorado, we have for years utilized a comparison of mountain climbing to that of labor to help both husband and wife know what to expect. In the early stages of labor the uterus is not working particularly hard or particularly often. Some labors skip this part or go through it quite rapidly to the more advanced type. If your wife is still in early labor (and let the doctor decide), there is no need for her to stay in bed.

Relaxation takes deep concentration and should be saved for later, more vigorous labor. We refer to this early labor as the gentle "foothills" that precede the higher mountains (see illustration). The uterus will contract occasionally as you stroll around with your wife. This results in a pressure feeling in her abdomen, back, or pelvis, and she may want to stop momentarily and lean over slightly. Husbands are good leaning posts, and during these few seconds she should bend over slightly, leaning on you, and

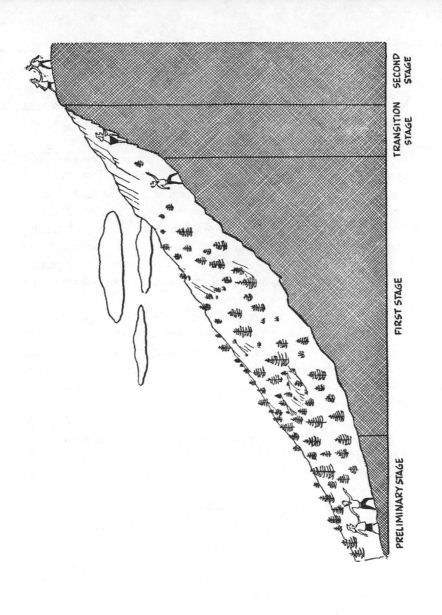

PRELIMINARY STAGE　　FIRST STAGE　　TRANSITION STAGE　　SECOND STAGE

lightly pant through parted lips until the contraction lets up—then you may amble on your way. There will probably be a lounge where you two may sit for a while during the foothill phase. Between contractions she will be in a conversational mood and chat with you, just as you two would were you climbing the foothills. There are occasional little steep parts where you must concentrate momentarily on the job of climbing. But there are regular declines and flat areas where again there is no particular need for concentration and idle chatter can be resumed. You will find your wife to be her usual good conversational self during these rhythmical phases. Your very presence is an overwhelming relief from boredom to your wife. She has nothing particularly to share, conversationally, with strangers (nurses, doctors, or otherwise), but she does with you.

As time goes on, the foothills become a little steeper, the inclines are longer, and the periods necessitating concentration become longer—the declines progressively get shorter and less frequent. These declines will gradually fade out as will her desire for carrying on conversation as the mountain gradually changes and becomes steeper.

After good, firm, regular uterine contractions are established, escort her back to the labor room, leisurely, for there is no hurry. The shortest labors, remember, occur in an atmosphere of peace and calmness, and your attitude and appearance can do much to promote this.

Now comes the more active part of your role as a coach. The uterine muscle is now getting down to real business, and your wife should now carefully imitate the other animals in her conduct during utering contractions. It really doesn't matter much what she does *between* uterine contractions, but it matters very much now what she does *during* them.

Let's get back to our observations of what nonhuman animals do in labor and carefully apply them to your wife's conduct now.

We have established needs for (1) a dimly lit room where

there is (2) quiet and privacy. Pick your hospital where family-centered principles are practiced (if you need help ask for it from the I.C.E.A.[2] until you find what you want). Now let's consider need (3), the need for physical comfort, as observed in the instinctive careful preparation of the "nest" by animals. How does this apply to your wife now, in labor?

First-stage labor in animals was briefly described as sleep imitation. Although they were not asleep, they looked like it and were positioned as in sleep. It behooves you as a husband, then, to have a good idea of how your big-tummied wife *positions* herself at home in her own bed while asleep. During the last few months of pregnancy you should make careful observations of her position in bed, the relationship of her arms, legs, etc., when she is deeply asleep. Try not to awaken her as you come in late from that long poker party with the boys, and carefully study her while she sleeps. She then presents the identical picture we want you as a labor coach to help her assume now in the hospital, by your careful guidance during her uterine contractions. This same position which she selected at home as being the most comfortable for her should be repeated at this stage of labor.

You will notice on the flat bed at home how she does not lie flat on her back—not at 3 A.M. during the last months of pregnancy. Some women may consciously start out the night lying on their backs due to ignorant misconceptions that they might hurt their baby if they lie on it. However, once their conscious mind is asleep, or partially so, they will subconsciously turn over on their sides, curl up in a ball, and adjust the pillow or pillows to the particular contours of their bodies. They usually sigh a deep, contented sigh as they achieve their particular position (this is strictly individual for every mother) and comfortably doze away.

In the last few months some mothers like to have a second pillow to support the top leg which is raised up higher than the

[2] International Childbirth Education Association, P.O. Box 5852, Milwaukee, Wisconsin 53220.

bottom leg to rotate the hips, allowing the heavy uterus to fall freely away from the mother and toward the bed. Have an extra pillow available in these later months of pregnancy and let your wife try out different combinations of support. *Let*, don't dictate. She will by experience work out her own positional pattern on her side. Having worked it out, you, as husband and coach, should be very familiar with it and now in first-stage labor, help her duplicate it in the hospital bed. If you need an additional pillow, ask for it. If it is wintertime and your wife mentions that her feet are cold (and some do even in summer), also ask for a hot water bottle, heating pad, or extra blanket. *Make her physically comfortable*. Know her little idiosyncrasies in advance. Such attentive care endears you to her.

Monotony and boredom constitute handicaps in the first stage of labor. This is the period when the forces of the uterine muscle must thin out and stretch the opening or "valve" through which the baby is to leave the uterus and enter the birth canal. This stage can be boring because the mother is required during the muscular action to simply "get out of the road" and let the action alone. This stage of do-nothingness is monotonous and takes great concentration on her part. Your very presence alone helps immensely, but there are things you can do also.

One of these things involves an occasional change of her position. At home on her flat bed there is only the one position for relaxation; curled up on her side. This involves an infinite number of variations in arm, leg, and pillow positions, differing from one person to another—e.g., some mothers put the lower arm underneath and along their backs, others snuggle this arm under the pillow, and so forth. You should be familiar with your wife's variations from your observations at home.

In the hospital, however, there is an additional position possible which your wife may find quite comfortable and which you cannot practice at home in advance. This is due to the adjustable nature of hospital beds compared with the one at home. I advise a husband whose wife is carrying twins or an extra large amount of salt water (and therefore larger distention of the abdomen) that he can win further endearment by renting a hospital bed during the last month for use at home.

The additional position for first-stage labor involves elevating both the upper and lower part of the hospital bed so your wife can assume a lounge chair or contour-like sprawl. She is neither sitting up nor lying down—rather in between these two. The two pillows are now used, folded up, under her arms and elbows to support them. Her knees should be sprawled, unladylike but mother-like, comfortably apart. The actual degree of elevation of either the upper or lower part of the bed should be, again, individually worked out by having *her* tell you what she prefers—after several trials. No pillow is usually used under the head, as the head can be raised further with the action of the bed if she wishes. Her arms and hands would otherwise fall awkwardly to her sides and interfere with relaxation unless pillows are folded to support the elbows and serve as arm rests (see illustration).

This position is based on the scientific principle that a group of muscles under tension cannot relax properly. All movable parts of the bone joints should be at the halfway station of the extent of their movement. Neither fully flexed (bent) nor fully extended (straightened), but rather at a happy medium of half and half. This you should consider as a coach in positioning your wife's wrists, elbows, shoulders, hips, knees, ankle joints, etc., as you adjust the bed and pillows.

As an illustration this point was brought to me forcibly when I was still experimenting early in my career with the group of nurses having their first babies. I was being ridiculed by some colleagues over the apparent lack of benefit of the relaxation teaching on one of our experimental patients. She was unable to achieve full relaxation and in general acted as if she had had no training at all in how to conduct herself during labor.

I had positioned her (pre-husband-participation days) in this contour or lounge chair position as part of the experiment. She had, up to then, been such a calm, capable person I was bewildered at her inability to relax fully during contractions. As I could see no reason for this, I asked her what *she thought* was interfering. She apologized over such a seemingly trivial thing— said she felt sort of silly—but the covers of the bed were bound down too tightly at the end of the bed and they held her feet down, forcibly pointing her toes, which made it impossible to relax.

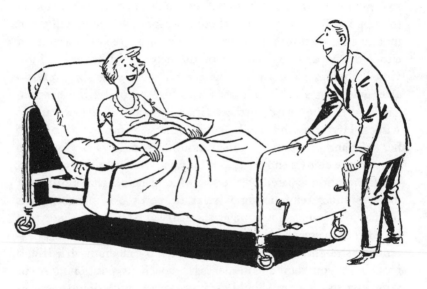

As soon as the problem was recognized and corrected by loosening the covers, she relaxed perfectly and performed magnificently for the rest of her labor. There is no detail too fine to be ignored in achieving the necessary degree of physical comfort required in labor. Don't hesitate to ask your wife for suggestions of what else you can do to make her comfortable.

Depending on the length of labor (and this is quite variable with every baby), your wife may want to alternate between this contour position and her old home one occasionally for variety. Try switching positions back and forth once in a while. Or if she prefers one position over the other and says so, fine, don't argue —only *she* knows how she feels.

We have seen some flexible-jointed slim ladies draw one or even both feet up and with their knees wide apart, rest their feet against the raised lower part of the bed. Since no two people are alike, we cannot dictate *exactly* how your wife should be positioned.

On a flat bed she should lie on her baby, never the reverse, her baby on her. Reassure her she cannot hurt a baby by lying on it (it's floating in salt water that equalizes any pressure), but it can jolly well hurt her by lying on her.

Never, never let your wife lie for any length of time flat on her back with her baby on top of her. Although this is necessary for short intervals to allow medical examinations, it is not only deucedly uncomfortably but also reduces blood flow to the heart and the kidneys and should *never* be a position in labor.

If you're ever out in the woods and find a pregnant animal lying flat on its back, balanced on its backbone, go get a spade and come back and bury it! No living pregnant animal would mistreat itself so.

I'll never forget the sight I beheld when I scouted a hospital to see if I wanted to bring my patients there, just before starting my practice. What I saw and heard made me run in terror and look elsewhere. A nurse was applying a restraining straight-jacket-like device on a laboring mother, strapping her flat on her back so she couldn't move. While adjusting the straps the nurse was verbally complaining to the patient: "Everytime I come to check you you're lying on your side. I told you to stay on your back so I can check your baby. Now we'll see if you mind," she added as she busily applied the restraining straps.

The mother was a wild-eyed medicated maniac, all conscious control long gone via medication. There was enough brain function left to know how much better it felt to lie on her side, and yet she was being deprived of that! In all fairness to the attending nurse, she had never been in labor herself and no one had ever informed her that a mother's position in labor makes a world of difference in how she feels. This is, I repeat, not the nurse's fault. It is rather the fault of the unawareness of the medical profession. Nurses follow doctors' orders.

If doubts exist in your mind whether position in labor affects how a woman feels, try it and see. You can momentarily experiment with your wife, just as I did many years ago with volunteer nurse mothers. You have nothing to lose but much to gain. To the best of your ability position your wife as has been outlined for first-stage labor. Now ask your wife to disobey any of our positional rules during a uterine contraction—e.g., lie flat on her back or in any awkward, strained position—and see what she says. Is there a difference? This challenge of "try it and see for yourself" we suggest after every itemized point of conduct which we have gleaned from observing animals in labor. Natural childbirth principles are not idly arrived at by armchair philosophical theory but are based upon observed facts.

We now come to need (4) observed in animals, physical relaxation of uninvolved muscles during labor. This represents the aspect technically most difficult for human imitation. Any stressful situation human beings encounter is met with the defense mechanism of muscular tension. Prior to the recognition of the stresses of life, human babies' muscles, when not in use, are automatically perfectly relaxed. As the stresses begin to accumulate (bowel training, personal neatness, making good grades, facing competition, keeping up with the Joneses, approaching parenthood, bossy mothers-in-law) the human being responds with tension. Inability to cope with stress is reflected in *excess* tension, e.g., tension headaches, spastic colons, nervous stomachs retaining gastric secretions too long due to muscular spasm until ulcers develop, and so forth.

In addition to the cluttered emotional-mental state of humans, which interferes with relaxation, there is a physical barrier to be overcome.

To perform any physical feat with grace and dexterity the human must practice and practice to achieve relaxation of uninvolved muscles. Such simple acts as running, jumping, even walking, are instinctively performed gracefully and automatically by nonhuman animals. Grace in physical action is a result of ability to keep the uninvolved muscles relaxed, an economy of muscular action. This does not mean we humans cannot achieve physical feats similar to animals. It means, rather, that we must recognize the human need for practice and physical conditioning of our muscles in the apparent absence of human instinct. Some people can run with the grace of a gazelle, swim like a fish, etc., but such abilities are acquired and maintained through practice.

Here, again, comes the factor of individuality. We are all different. Some humans need far more practice than others to achieve the same physical goals. This, topped by the heavy human overlay of emotional factors, creates quite a complex picture.

To the repeated inquiry "Do you think every woman can learn to do natural childbirth?" I counter with another question. Do you think every woman in the absence of physical abnormalities can be taught to swim? They are both acts instinctively performed by animals. We have to contend with individual variations again. Some humans take to water like ducks, others are rigid and fearful of water. The human emotional factor is important. An inexperienced woman who has been thrown into deep water against her wishes and nearly drowned is the rest of her life a very real challenge to a swimming instructor. The very thought or sight of water makes her *rigid* with fear. Nevertheless with patient reassurance and step-by-step training, even she can still be taught to swim.

Similarly, some women take to natural childbirth with ease and grace and a minimum of coaching. Others, especially if they have had a frightening experience in childbirth previously, take a lot more practice and more patient, reassuring coaching. Both types can reach the same success; the coaching technique is different.

The farm girl who has known only the peace and happiness of animal births is an easy coaching case (e.g., the sheep rancher cited previously). I get much more personal satisfaction out of the challenge of high-strung "nervous" patients who, when we first meet them, are scared to death to have a baby. Is there such a thing as a woman who is too nervous and high-strung to utilize natural childbirth? Good heavens, this is the type who, above all others, *needs* natural childbirth. I have an ego-deflating feeling that the female sheep rancher could have performed perfectly well on the range without having ever been near a doctor.

Perhaps you recall reading the fascinating story by the charming actress Julie Harris[3] on the birth of her first baby? Her doctor dismissed natural childbirth as not applicable in her case because as an actress she was too nervous and high-strung.

She returned home in despair and tears to report this to her husband. He, however, had read up on natural childbirth and it was obvious to him that the doctor had not. The husband indignantly maintained this wasn't true and he would teach her himself! He proceeded to work with his wife at home, practicing the principles with her in careful preparation for the birth. He then accompanied her to the hospital and served as her coach. Can you think of a better coach than an attentive, educated, loving husband? Result: she gave birth to the baby rapidly and joyfully before the doctor got there! When, during the labor, the attending nurses attempted to send the husband-coach away, Julie vehemently stated, "When he leaves, I leave." I think the attendants got the message: she meant business. He was essential to the task at hand and she knew it.

Your wife can be shown the principles of relaxation and she can be taught the consciousness of her muscles' state of tension in prenatal classes under the supervision of experienced teachers. Being a human animal, however, she needs to practice these principles at home daily in order to perfect them. This you can

[3] "I Was Afraid to Have a Baby," *Reader's Digest*, April 1957, condensed from *McCall's*, December 1956.

help her do. A suggested time is just before retiring for the night as a prelude to sleep. This serves a double purpose: It establishes her self-confidence in her physical relaxation ability, and it is an aid to peaceful slumber.

We have found the following step-by-step pattern of deliberate awareness of "letting go" muscle tension in definite body areas, one after the other, to be most effective. Starting from the top down, relaxing the forehead, eyelids, face muscles, jaw, neck, shoulders, arm muscles, chest, abdomen, hips, thighs, legs, and feet. This step-like progression should be accompanied with a gentle, light touch of the various areas, stroking lightly with the finger tips. The husband coach should give verbal suggestions of relaxation in a diminishing volume of voice, ending with nearly a whisper. Test your wife's ability by gently lifting and dropping her hand, gently shaking her foot or ankle, gently rolling her head from side to side to make her aware of any residual neck tension. Her position during this practice at home should be her individual sleep position on her side, which you have previously arrived at by observing her during deep sleep.

Do not have her try to maintain this deep conscious relaxation for long intervals. This is practically impossible over long periods, and besides the uterine muscle hardly ever contracts for more than one minute. Interrupt your practice at home with stretch sessions and low back rubs.

The baby box is a heavy organ and is fastened to the mother only in the low back area by a set of muscles called the uterosacrals, going from the uterus to the sacrum or "saddle" area. This is the curved area of the low back where, if your wife will pardon my illustration, the saddle would be placed on a horse. Rub this area firmly and slowly with the heel of your hand. Lubricate the skin with talcum powder or cold cream to allow your hand to slide freely. She'll probably murmur approval—it feels good! These muscles get tired carrying babies around all day; massage them firmly at bedtime. Now at an agreed signal, imagine the return of another uterine contraction and for one minute teach her to carefully relax. Warm relaxation takes the place of cold tension as the tension goes down and out, from top to bottom, face to feet, systematically, deliberately.

Now we come to a facet of human relaxation which is inescapable. The relationship of mind-body, or the psycho-somatic nature of humans. The mind and body are interacting, one helping or hindering the other. It is probably impossible to relax the body completely if the mind is under tension. Vice versa, it is impossible to relax the mind completely if the body is under tension. This is observed also in animals in their need to concentrate during labor and the temporary viciousness of laboring animals if this concentration is disrupted in any way.

We have been stressing deliberate "do nothingness" of the body during uterine contractions. Can you similarly relax the mind, make it go blank and "think nothingness"? No! it can't be done. It's like trying not to think of an elephant. If you can't think of nothing during moments of concentrated physical relaxation, then you must think of something. What should your wife think about, how should she occupy her mind while relaxing her body? Her mother-in-law problem? The fight with the neighbors? The bills yet unpaid? Hardly conducive to relaxation! No, she should select the earliest and most pleasant memory from her childhood and deliberately dwell on this happy little experience. She should relive it in all its pleasant aspects, utilizing every known sensory function in her recall—sights, sounds, fragrances, touch, taste—to make it more real. Early childhood states of trust and total dependence on others were accompanied then by automatic physical relaxation—test the muscular relaxation of sleeping children. Recalling and reliving happy days in the mind's eye during uterine contractions helps her to dissociate from the pulling feeling in her back and lower abdomen. It is also a wonderful prelude to sleep for her and, incidentally, you. It is an automatic turning off of the mental worries, doubts, and frustrations which beset the day, to allow both the mind and body to relax as efficiently as it did in early childhood—you *can* sleep "like a baby" if you put your mind to it.

Now such mental focusing of attention or mental control takes careful concentration on the part of your wife. This is more easily achieved in familiar surroundings with familiar sounds. The maternity ward of a hospital, even the better ones, tends to be distracting. Some have installed background music to help achieve relaxation. This is all right as far as it goes; it's a step in the right direction, but we have found by actual experience that there is a "background music" that beats all others and there is no substitute for it. It is the familiar beloved voice of a husband, a lover gently, softly, endearingly whispering in his sweetheart's ear that same line of love gobbledygook that was instrumental in starting the whole business of babies in the first place! This is where you come in as a husband, and, by heaven, you're the only one who can play this role. Other instructors can teach physical relaxation, but it takes a lover to teach true mental relaxation.

Early in my tumultuous career of getting hospital administrators to allow husbands throughout labor I was capitalizing on one particular husband being with his wife because he was a doctor, an M.D., and therefore was allowed back in "no man's land." After the birth was completed I had the radiant mother tell the superintendent her reaction to natural childbirth.

I asked her in his presence if she had really wanted her husband with her. She unhesitatingly stated, "Oh, I couldn't have gotten along without him." I then asked if this was because of his being a doctor. She replied, "No, that had nothing to do with it. I needed him because he is my lover, not my doctor."

Play the lover role, then, during the glorious climax to your act of love—the birth of your baby.

Superficially you may think such details quite trite, but experience has taught us to bring food trays into the labor room for the husband as well as the wife, as we have seen uncontrolled panic take the place of calm cooperation when we sent the husband out, even for a moment, to get a bite to eat. Family-centered hospitals will knowingly take this into consideration.

Your wife will peacefully relive her happy childhood scene undisturbed by the forces of the uterine contraction (or a boiler factory) if she has that familiar, loved background music of your voice and your presence to reassure and encourage her. She feels secure in your presence—or she wouldn't have married you in the first place.

The irreplaceability of a husband as a labor coach was illustrated just the other day by an incident. I arrived in the labor room to do the initial check on one of our patients in labor. She had come in during busy office hours and since she was still in early labor, I had seen a few more patients in our nearby office before stopping in to see her. Shortly after I entered the room a uterine contraction began. I observed facial tension and rather poor abdominal breathing, and started fussing over these departures from what she had been taught. Her husband rose from his chair at her side and much to my delight laid a reassuring hand on my shoulder and said, "Don't worry, Doc, she does just fine when you're not here." I couldn't help laughing with them at the interfering element of my presence. To such efficient teamwork I merely reminded her if she felt like pushing (second stage), to push on two things—the hospital signal button first and her bottom second, at least to let me know when the baby was coming so I could build up my ego by catching it. I went back to the office to see waiting patients, thinking how a few hours spent in evening classes teaching husbands to be labor coaches paid off so well in saving doctors' and nurses' time in the course of labor.

We have discussed at some length the beneficial effect on the mother (and doctor!) of having a husband with his wife during first-stage labor. Now, what of the effect on the husband? I wish every reader could ask that question of a husband who has known the anxious, lonely vigil of pacing the waiting room floor with a previous baby and then received training and coached his wife during labor with a subsequent birth. Seek such men out and ask them, if you have the opportunity. They'll talk your arm off on the benefits of being a participant. I routinely ask the husband after the birth is completed if he'd rather have been out in the waiting room during the labor. I get many explosive comments—"Not on your life," "I'd have gone crazy out there," etc.

Now back to our comparison of how animals conduct themselves in labor and how you can teach your wife to do likewise. No. 5 is the need for controlled breathing. If you recall, in first-stage labor we observed animals breathing the same way as they do when asleep—with their abdomen. Because labor is what the term implies, hard work, the depth and rapidity of breathing will vary with the length and strength of the uterine contraction. Your wife should also breathe in the same fashion she does when deeply asleep. However, her depth and rate of breathing will gradually increase as the labor progresses.

Sleep breathing is technically diaphragmatic breathing. Because the abdomen is visible and the diaphragm is not, we usually refer to it as abdominal breathing. In a state of relaxation her abdomen will rise and fall as her diaphragm goes down (inspiration) and up (expiration). Her diaphragm may be compared to the piston in an air pump—as it descends it pulls air in, as the piston rises it pushes the air out. You cannot see the diaphragm working, as it is a hidden muscle, domelike in shape, separating the abdominal cavity from the chest cavity. As it descends the abdomen must necessarily rise. As the diaphragm rises the abdomen will fall back down. If a mother should inadvertently hold her abdomen rigid, then diaphragmatic action is impossible and she must then expand her rib cage to allow air to enter her chest. A rigidly held abdomen also interferes with the dome of the uterus going forward during contraction to allow its full force to act directly against the cervix.

Here's where husbands again prove their usefulness. When the uterine muscle contracts, it is directly under the abdominal muscle, and unless a mother exercises self-control she will tend to tighten her abdominal muscle along with the uterine muscle. To her, especially with her eyes closed, she can't *see* the difference, and because of the close proximity of the two muscles she can't *feel* the difference. Now you as an "outsider" can see the difference, and if you will lightly place your hand on her abdomen you can also *feel* the difference. In other words you can tell what she is doing and she can't. Guide her and coach her until you see and feel that she is breathing properly—during a contraction. Under your guidance, she will learn to "bulge" her abdomen out actively, deliberately, with each inspiration and then let go and rhythmically let her abdomen drop back down with expiration. The weight of your hand laid lightly on her abdomen serves as a guide. This can be further expedited if you will give her abdomen a gentle nudge or tap at the beginning of inspiration when it is time to bulge actively. She will feel the rhythm of giving your hand a ride on the waves, up and down, or a sensation that her abdomen is an accordion and she is rhythmically opening and closing it to affect the coming and going of air. Should she get mixed up and hold her abdomen down, necessitating expanding her rib cage, gently correct this by verbal and touch guidance.

This type of coaching is most easily achieved in the propped-up contour chair position, as you are better able to observe the movements of the abdomen. It is usually automatically done in the side position as in sleep at home. However, if she has trouble catching on to the rhythm, utilize the "contour chair" until her confusion is cleared up. You can then lower the bed and have her curl up on her side again. Slip your hand on her abdomen while she's on her side and resume the nudge or tap signal with each inhalation—rhythmically.

Abdominal or diaphragmatic breathing can be rehearsed at home during the course of pregnancy. A semi-propped-up position on the davenport or bed, using a pillow or rolled blanket underneath the knees, to simulate the hospital bed in a cranked-up position will probably prove most convenient. The commercial contour or lounge chair could also be used. Both you and your wife will find this deliberate breathing rather simple to perform before the onset of labor. The effect of the uterine contraction in labor may be at first confusing to your wife. She may get the bewildering feeling that the uterine muscle is her abdominal muscle. Of course this isn't so—she has the same set of abdominal breathing muscles, capable of being utilized for such, whether the uterine muscle is contracting or not. The two groups are separate and work independently of each other, but she needs your guidance and objective analysis to help her distinguish between the two.

The last observation of instinctive conduct (No. 6) is the need for closed eyes during first-stage labor.

Again, this is probably relevant to the simple need to exclude visual distractions to allow concentration. It is just as necessary with your wife as it is with the cat having kittens or the dog having pups. She must literally mind her own business and pay total attention to what she is doing (relaxation and abdominal breathing). Her labor is all-encompassing and requires her full span of mental and physical powers.

In early labor she will only close her eyes during the actual time her uterus is contracting. As the "mountain gets steeper," requiring more and more of her attention, she will tend to keep her eyes closed even between contractions in order not to allow any distractions. In this phase do not attempt to draw her into the idle conversation which she so readily and cheerfully entered into during the foothills phase. Do not hold her hand or make any physical contacts that would distract her attention. Such advances on your part are motivated by noble thoughts and a desire to let her know of your intentions, but because they are distracting her from her work she may, like the other animal mothers, snap at you—verbally of course. I had trouble in my early career of not properly preparing husbands for this possibility and had several get their feelings hurt. They were only trying to help but didn't realize they were actually hindering their wives. I had to reassure them that this did not reflect alteration of love for them —this is evident even in animals. They may warn disturbing masters by snapping during labor, but their affection is unaltered when the job is done.

Along with the sleep imitation aspect and the closed eyes I will comment on another facial characteristic that is probably the only true total muscle relaxation—mouth dropping open. Your observation of your wife deeply asleep will reveal parted lips and mouth breathing. A moment's reflection by any person will bring to mind the phenomenon of a rather awful taste in one's mouth upon awakening in the morning. It represents simply the drying-out effect of breathing through one's mouth during deep relaxed sleep. This is the largest and therefore easiest route for air to pass—it takes effort to force air through the narrower nasal passages—and in deep sleep the body is economizing on effort. We have often threatened, jokingly, to put a "bulldog" clothespin on the nose of any mother we catch breathing through her nose in labor. It simply isn't done! All labor involves efficient air exchange, and good athletes breathe through their *mouths*. Labor also produces the morning taste in the mouth, which makes the complimentary iced orange juice given to all natural childbirth mothers (and fathers, if they're there) a very pleasant experience.

Laughter is the one great distinguishing characteristic in natural-birth rooms, and I recall one patient who had us all laughing at the moment of birth, including, I assure you, her husband. It was her sixth child in practically as many years and all by this method. She firmly maintained that the only reason she got pregnant so often was to get this glass of iced orange juice because it was the best drink she had ever tasted.

When the late Dr. Grantly Dick-Read of England honored us with a visit several years ago he made a twinkly-eyed comment that they would never allow this concept in his country—at birth they gave "hot tea with plenty of 'sugah'!"

Transition Stage

The first stage of labor is arbitrarily defined as the period of cervical dilatation. The last portion of this stage—from about 8 centimeters dilatation in first-baby labors, and 6 centimeters to complete dilatation (10 cm.) in women who have previously borne children—has been given a special category by itself known as the "transition stage."

In animals we observed that prior to this stage they may get up and move about, change position, turn around, etc. In transition stage they settle down and stay in one preferred position and discontinue any extra movements. They also concentrate deeply on what they are doing and are quite uncommunicative. They will very definitely snap crossly at anyone or anything that tends to disturb their concentration during this stage.

The same is necessarily true of human mothers. This is the steepest part of the mountain (see illustration on page 31) and there is great need to pay constant attention to what one is doing. You will find your wife completely uncommunicative during this period. No more idle chatter between contractions. The interval between contractions has now diminished until your wife seems to think there is no interval at all—one contraction seems to follow closely upon the other. Don't try to engage in conversation. Do not attempt hand holding or any other "extra" maneuver during this period—unless she requests it. She may not want the intermittent back rubs now; there may not be time enough between uterine contractions, and your ministrations that were so gratefully received earlier will now only serve to disturb her concentration on relaxation, as the contractions are nearly continuous.

Continue the low-voiced, gentle, monotonous talking, now nearly whispering, in her ear. Continue the gentle pressure of your hand on her abdomen to guide her breathing—but no "extras" now.

What subjective feelings is your wife experiencing? She has a progressively increasing pressure feeling in her lower abdomen, back, and "bottom." Her birth canal is gradually filling up with descent of the presenting part (that part coming first) of the baby, usually the baby's head. Because of the proximity of the rectum behind the birth canal (it's truly a next-door neighbor) even though it has been efficiently emptied by the enema in early labor it now feels fuller and fuller. One patient described the sensation as feeling "constipateder and constipateder" as time goes on. Even before the cervix has completely opened, the baby gets lower and lower. This sensation your wife should interpret as progress. She needs to have been reassured in advance that such progressive pressure feelings mean she's getting somewhere and that such pressure is beneficial to both baby and bottom (mother's). Soon we'll be over the hump of the mountain to the more gentle plateau that just precedes completion, and that glorious achievement will soon be realized.

The crescendo action of the uterus gives your wife very little time to gather her wits or self-control between contractions. She may tend to get little panicky feelings because of this. Reassure her in a firm voice if she tends to lose self-control. Get the train back on the tracks if she tends to break the rhythm of what she has been doing. I think the most encouraging comment you can make is, "We'll be seeing our baby soon" or "We'll soon know if it's a boy or a girl." Take her mind off herself and on to the joy of seeing the baby. If your reassurance is not effective, ask for help from the doctor—he is familiar with the panicky feeling of transition stage and can assist you in reassuring your wife. The calm patient will proudly recognize that the efficient close contractions, the increasing pressure in her baby box means "Now we're getting somewhere." Your wife can tell by the tendency she will feel to push or bear down that the actual passage of the baby (second stage) is imminent now. She will tend to be confused whether she should push now with her contractions. Old-timers—experienced natural childbirth mothers who have consciously given birth previously—know jolly well when it's pushing time, and as a doctor I have learned it is a waste of time to check them (feel the cervix either vaginally or rectally); they know. However, if this is your wife's first child or first one by natural childbirth, she should be checked by the attending doctor or nurse to be sure the cervix is fully dilated. This is compared to being sure the door is fully open before you push the car out of the garage. If your wife gets the urge to push and the doctor or nurse is not there at the moment summon them by the signal bell. It may be confusing to your wife as to whether it is truly pushing time or not. If the examination shows the cervix is not completely dilated, there would be no point in pushing quite yet—it wouldn't do any harm but would be ineffectual. She should then be encouraged to continue her relaxation phase and her deep, rhythmical, free breathing for just a while longer until the door is completely open. Encourage her that true pushing time will really be here shortly—as it will be if she will relax and breathe deeply and freely just a little longer.

In women having their first baby the transition stage usually lasts about one hour. For those who have had previous babies it may be only a momentary phase and pass so quickly as to be indistinguishable. In either case it is the shortest phase of labor, and your wife should be made cognizant of this *before* she enters labor. Then she will recognize it as the acme of accomplishment which ushers in the most satisfactory and rewarding of all stages, the part where the mother gets to "do something"—push—with her uterine contraction. It is far simpler to do something than to do nothing.

5

Second-Stage Labor and Birth

Squatting and Pushing

THE STEEPEST PART of the mountain has been climbed. Now you and your wife have gone over the hump and are traversing the more gradual plateau that precedes the summit. You can see the goal ahead. You will very soon get that magnificent view (of your baby) that your efforts have been directed toward. I pray for the day when all hospitals will have a natural childbirth wing set aside so that all husbands can bring cameras on their trip and take a picture of this magnificent view. Because of the total absence of anesthetists and gas machines in natural-birth rooms our hospital has allowed "daddy pictures" at birth ever since we introduced natural childbirth. These photos, even though amateurishly taken by husbands enrich the baby book—vividly proving to the growing child forever after the joy and happiness his birth brought to his mother and father. How many psychoses or personality deviations of later life have been based on a feeling of rejection—of not having been wanted in the first place?

Grateful husbands have given us copies of these pictures to be used in introducing the concepts of natural childbirth to the bewildered, frightened, inexperienced parents-to-be. When his wife is that happy, that radiantly beautiful at the moment of birth,

52

why should a husband not share the experience? Ask your doctor to show you some of these pictures and study them with your wife. They are like picture post cards taken of the view at the summit of a mountain by experienced climbers. But they, are only pictures of others' experiences. How much more meaningful will it be for you and your wife to actually climb the mountain and see for yourself.

These are the thoughts you can transmit to your wife now that she has achieved the plateau that precedes the summit—the pushing stage, the last stage, of labor, the stage just before you see and hear your baby.

In order that you manage this stage properly let's make sure that you understand it completely. Through knowledge and understanding we achieve proper performance. Let's go back to our instructors—the cat having kittens, the dog having pups, etc.—and carefully observe their actions so that we may then apply them to ours.

Up to now the animal has carefully imitated sleep—in location, position, appearance, breathing, etc. When the mother animal's cervix completely opens, allowing the baby to slip out of the uterus down into the birth canal (vagina), the baby pushes against a set of muscles called the levator ani group. This pressure sets up a reflex nearly identical to that set up by peristaltic movements of the colon pushing its contents down into the lower rectum, producing the urgency to have a bowel movement.

I do not know why the Creator unaesthetically put the baby door in this particular location—between the bladder and the rectum. It has necessitated a very unladylike but definitely mother-like position known as squatting to perform the act of giving birth. Whether we like it or not, the act of emptying the baby box is mechanically identical to emptying the rectum. As a man I will never know what it actually feels like having a baby. Being very interested in subjectively preparing mothers-to-be so they will know in advance what it feels like, I have asked this question, by questionnaire and verbally, of thousands of experienced natural childbirth mothers, whose clear minds, unclouded by medication, know perfectly well what it feels like. I have always received the same answer: "It feels like having a big bowel movement."

We noticed in the animal mothers that when the cervix dilates completely and the baby descends against this set of muscles the animals change automatically from sleep imitation to "having a bowel movement" action. That is, they arch their backs, hold their breath and make expulsive grunting noises. They follow the urge or signal given by the descent of the baby with appropriate action.

This natural urge is also followed automatically by even untrained human mothers. We refer to it as the "gotta go" urge, or in some surprised, untrained mothers who acted involuntarily, the "Oh my gosh, I just did" action. I recall seeing a mother in consultation because her cervix hadn't completely dilated. It had opened to 8 centimeters and remained there for quite a long time without progressing. Probably as a result of the calming influence of the specialist being introduced and the verbal exchange of reassuring pleasantries while I was donning a sterile glove to examine her, she became relaxed enough to allow the baby's head to slip through the cervix. I never did do the examination. I didn't have to. The young mother got this startled look on her face, involuntarily held her breath for a moment, and apologizing profusely, begged me not to pull the sheet down to examine her until the nurse had cleaned her up because she had "just done something right in bed that I haven't done since I was a baby!" She was gently reminded that her rectum was completely emptied earlier by the enema and that the feeling was actually due to the descent of the baby. I assured her that she didn't need the examination now, that it was obvious her cervix had just finished dilating, and coached her how to squat, hold her breath, and more efficiently do what she had just inadvertently partially done—push her baby down. Her gratitude was heart-warming.

Animals in second-stage labor, then, act, look, and breathe as though they are having a bowel movement. So what should your wife do after her cervix is completely open and the baby begins to slip through? She should do the same thing. Now, here again, we run into the minor structural differences between humans and animals. They are minor but important. You will have made a careful study of how your wife conducts herself in sleep for management of the first-stage labor. Must you now make a similar study in the bathroom and see how your wife manages a bowel movement? Definitely not. For two reasons. One is she just might resent such invasion of her privacy, and the other reason is she's not conducting herself correctly there anyway. This isn't her fault, it's the fault of so-called civilization and the invention of toilet stools. These gadgets designed erroneously to make it easier for human beings have probably been instrumental in keeping proctologists (rectal specialists) in business. This point was brought to my mind rather emphatically early in my specialty training by having made the acquaintance of a young doctor from India who had come to this country and to the same university for postgraduate specialty training. I found him a fascinating chap and we became close friends. One day we entered the men's rest room together and to my amazement he climbed up on the American toilet with his feet on the lid and assumed the squatting position. At my sarcastic jibes he countered with the statement that in his country people properly squatted to move their bowels and that in his medical training in India he had not observed hemorrhoids; he had had to come to my country to find these abnormalities. We got into a heated discussion of what constituted civilization. I frankly didn't believe his statement that the bathroom facilities in his lavish home in India consisted of openings on the level floor over which one squatted. I'm sure his mother in India was most bewildered when she received a request in his next letter that she photograph their bathroom and send the picture along, but she obligingly did so and thus helped to educate this backward foreigner.

I grudgingly came to the conclusion that he was right. The human body is so designed that the farther apart and the farther back the legs go the less flesh there is in the way of obstructing the downward passage of a bowel movement or a baby! A moment's serious thought would serve to illustrate this in contemplating children, prior to their introduction to toilet stools. I was giving a prenatal class a few years ago and covering this particular subject. We keep this introductory class as informal as possible. While I was talking one of the restless little toddler children in the group, diaper clad and not toilet trained, was ambling in front of me. Just at this appropriate moment the child stopped, squatted perfectly, held its breath, got red in the face as it, obvious to all, had a bowel movement in its diaper. There couldn't have been a better illustration of my topic and it gained a round of applause from the group.

No, labor coach, the bathroom fixture confuses the principles. Rather, let us visualize the proper position your wife should assume based upon observation of children, people of the Orient, or you yourself on a hunting trip out in the woods with no toilet stools around. This position is the squatting position and by now should be very familiar to both you and your wife as you have coached her to perform it many times in her household duties during pregnancy. (See Chapter 6.)

If the attending doctor or nurse has found by examination that the cervix is open—or if your wife is experienced on the subjective manifestations of labor and knows on her own that this is truly pushing time—then you should coach her to assume this full squatting position. From her standpoint it could more easily be done on the floor, as at home during her pregnancy. However, this is inconvenient for the attendants who need to cleanse, examine and observe, etc.

In the latter portion of first stage and during transition stage most mothers find the contour chair, propped-up position most comfortable. A few mothers may still be on their sides when the cervix opens completely. Although it is true that the mother's legs could be drawn back and apart, and she could hump her back while on her side and give birth to her baby (used successfully in home deliveries and flat beds), hospital labor beds can be cranked up in the semi-sitting position and we have found this quite convenient for squatting in second stage.

If your wife is not already in the contour chair position, we suggest you crank the bed up and have her assume it. It provides a restful position between contractions in second stage. During contractions she should arch her back, pulling her head and shoulders forward (trying to peer over her pregnant tummy) by drawing her knees back and apart with her arm muscles. Her elbows should be thrust out and each wrist and forearm securely locked under her knees. In this position during her downward pushing she should let her leg muscles be completely relaxed as she pulls with her arms. This allows her thighs to get farther and farther apart and back, serving to get the flesh between her legs (the inner upper part of her thighs) out of the way of the baby so it can descend. This action literally serves to open the baby door.

This can be done in the labor room bed or on the delivery room table. It helps greatly if the former is propped up like a contour chair, and if the latter is tilted with the head up and the foot downward. The degree of tilt should be nearly to the point of letting the mother slide down, nearly a 45-degree angle. If your doctor is not oriented to natural childbirth principles, make the request during pregnancy to have the delivery room table tilted downward.

The hospital custom where anesthetics are used is to tilt the table with the *head* down, bottom up. This is to attempt to make vomitus or secretions from the nose and mouth drain by gravity away from the air opening in mothers who are put to sleep. Natural childbirth mothers find this upside down position ridiculous and a hindrance to conscious expulsion of the baby. They say it's like trying to have a B.M. using a bedpan in a flat bed, trying to go uphill to do a downhill job.

Because the delivery room table is usually an unadjustable flat affair we utilize two pillows—one under the mother's shoulders, one under her head for support. As she pushes with contractions you as a coach can help immeasurably by pushing the pillows so that they follow her arching back forward. If you are fortunate enough to have a Fitzhugh back support adapter on the table, this will not be necessary. Most hospitals have yet to acquire these excellent supports, so that the adjustable back support remains an educated, pillow-adjusting husband.

If this is your wife's first baby there will be time enough in second stage to perform for a while in the labor room bed. If this is not her first baby she will probably be moved to the delivery (birth) room shortly after reaching second stage, or some doctors may even want her moved there before she starts pushing, if she has had several previous babies. Let your doctor decide.

We have covered the *position* of second-stage labor in the imitation of bowel movement action. Whereas we had six points of performance to follow in first-stage labor, we have only three in the simple action of second stage. The first is position, squatting; the second is breath holding.

Breath Control

You will note that anyone moving his bowels does so by holding his breath during the act. Your wife, then, should be an efficient breath holder during her uterine contractions in second-stage labor. Her breath control now is totally different from first stage. For the two stages of labor the conduct is very different indeed. In order for her to hold her breath during the entire length of the uterine contraction—or as much of it as she can—she is going to need all the breath her lungs can hold. Therefore instead of the gentle abdominal breaths of the first stage she should be encouraged now to breathe large, deep chest breaths, opening her rib cage to its fullest diameter to accommodate as much air as possible. I think a good comparison for our term "athletic breathing" in second stage is an underwater swimming race. The swimmer plans to exert his energies for as long as possible on one breath, under water, to see who can swim the farthest. Whoever wins the race will be dependent upon how thoroughly he fills his lungs with air before he is called upon to hold it.

In quiet breathing there is a lot of unused stale reserve air present. This stale air must be "washed out" by deeply inhaling and exhaling first. The efficient swimmer would fill up completely, empty out completely several times to rid the lungs of stale air, and completely replace with fresh. When your wife feels her uterine contraction beginning she should calmly open her chest and inhale as fully as possible three times. The first two lungfuls should be completely emptied out by totally exhaling. The third big breath is the one she should hold, at the height of inspiration, with her lungs fully filled with fresh air. She should calmly hold this full breath and simultaneoulsy hump over, chin on chest, put her arms under her knees, and, elbows out sideways, pull with strong arm action until her limp, relaxed legs come completely back and apart as far as they can. When she has held this breath as long as she comfortably can (there is no need to act heroic and try to hold beyond comfort), she should exhale completely. If, at this time, the uterine contraction is still present, she should immediately *inhale* completely and hold this second time as long as the breath holds out. She should then exhale again completely, emptying all of the air, and in the rare instance that the uterus is still working, she could repeat another big inhalation and hold this—until the contraction lets up. All breathing is open-mouthed with an open, relaxed throat.

During the rest periods between contractions she should let her legs slip back on the elevated foot of the bed, or if she is on a flat delivery room table, into the metal troughs provided for supporting the legs during rest periods. One of the fundamentals for the consciously cooperating mother is that she should *never* be restricted in any way. Her arms and legs should not be bound down by leather straps or held in any position against her will as are those of uncooperative medicated patients. This is a *must* that should be clearly understood and agreed upon in advance by the doctor and his attendants.

Pushing

The third point of performance for your wife in the second-stage of labor is the muscular action of pushing. Again, unaesthetic as it may be, this muscular action is identical in performance to that of being constipated and squatting out in the woods with the firm determination of moving one's bowels. Breaking down the details of action, it involves downward action of the abdominal muscles while holding the diaphragm-breathing muscle immobile, via breath holding, so that the increase in intra-abdominal pressure is directed downward and out the flexible opening of the vagina. Simultaneously this muscle-surrounded aperture, the vagina, should be deliberately opened by consciously relaxing the circular, or sphincter, muscles which surround it. These circular muscles when tightened tend to draw the vagina upward and closed. When relaxed the vagina descends downward and open.

For unknown reasons which again only the Creator can clear up, this set of muscles is also part of and controlled by the same muscles which open or close the bladder (in front) and the rectum (in back). Anatomically this is a single muscle divided into three component parts in women. It is called the pubococcygeus muscle, as it passes from the pubic (in front) to the coccygeal bone (behind). However, it has circular parts which surround the urethra (bladder opening) in front, vagina in the middle, and anal sphincter (rectal opening) in the back

For simplicity and out of respect for Dr. Kegel who first described its importance[1] we refer to this muscle as the Kegel muscle and put great emphasis on its utilization.

While your wife is pushing down she should deliberately relax this muscle at the same time that she is tightening her abdominal and arm muscles. The purpose is, of course, to aid in opening the vagina for the passage of the baby. You, as a coach, can help her by verbally reminding her as she pushes to try to urinate and try to move her bowels, or "Kegel relax," as she pushes. A woman who holds back by tightening this muscle for fear she might release urine or bowel movement is also holding back her baby, and instead of pushing the baby down and out is merely playing tug of war with her own sets of muscles and is ineffectually squeezing the baby.

We have tried discontinuing the routine enema given as part of the "prep" on admission in labor. I doubt very much whether it is necessary, actually, from a physical standpoint. However, from a psychological standpoint we found it to be very helpful in most cases. We find our mothers push down more effectively if they know their rectum is empty. They seem to have a psychological hesitancy to move their bowels in this exposed position, probably a carry-over from childhood toilet training. When we encourage them to go ahead and try to move their bowels, with the further reassurance that they actually can't due to the thorough enema they had, then they cooperate much better. The same thing seems to hold for emptying the bladder. If they have had the enema, in the process of expelling it they automatically empty their bladders (it's the same muscle control). We do not catheterize natural childbirth mothers and we noticed a tendency, when they had not had an enema, to hold back in second stage for fear they would release urine. With emptied bladders after an enema they did not hesitate to "Kegel relax." As a natural childbirth doctor, let me reassure all mothers: if in the act of pushing we do not observe some small passage of urine or actual opening

[1] A. H. Kegel, "The Non-Surgical Treatment of Genital Relaxation," *Ann. West. Med. & Surg.* 2:213-216, May 1948.

of the rectum, we tend to get upset and fussy, not the other way around.

Another of the many benefits of natural childbirth is the paucity of bladder problems afterward. There is no need for catheters before, during, or after the *birth* of a baby, only from the *delivery* of a baby. No matter how careful and sterile the technique of catheterization, it is an undignified, miserable feeling, traumatizing to some degree the urinary passageway as well as introducing existing bacteria from the outside to the inside of the bladder.

The other day a new obstetrical patient who had had both previous babies by anesthetics was told that with natural childbirth she could go home with her baby any time she wished after two hours from birth (if she breast fed). She asked if we did house calls to catheterize our patients! Such a possibility had never occurred to us—it had never been needed. Mothers who can empty their vaginas themselves can certainly empty their bladders themselves.

We encourage the husband to encourage his wife to deliberately wet the bed while pushing. We joke to the couples that, after all, the husband pays for the laundry here and the wife doesn't have to rinse out a thing during her visit. The "open door policy" must prevail during pushing, and in order to get one door to open all three must be opened. Why, I don't know; just take it the way it comes.

We men can never know what it feels like to have a baby. The most thorough and intelligent description I ever read, however, is in Helen Wessel's brilliant book, *Natural Childbirth and the Christian Family*. She knows the *subjective* feelings and describes them vividly.

As an observer at many births let me share with you my *objective* observations so that you will have a deeper understanding when you are privileged to be present.

In second-stage labor, before the baby is actually coming outside the mother's body, that is, during its descent down through the internal portions of the birth canal, your wife's face will have about the same appearance as that of a piano mover who is intermittently called upon to lift a heavy piano, hold it for a minute, then set it down, rest and chat for a few minutes, then lift it up and hold it some more. Her face will get a reddish color during this breath-holding (as did the little toddler's at the prenatal class), and her features will be contorted in the same way that piano movers' are—with effort, not pain. Please, please do not confuse these two.

I recall a "stubborn Dutchman," as his wife referred to him, who was very skeptical over his active role. He actually wanted no part of being a participant in the birth. Out of due respect to our many wonderful Dutch-descended patients, he had reasons. Darn good reasons. When I noticed his reluctance to attend classes preparing him as a coach, I inquired why.

His frank answer was revealing, "Doc, I sat out in that waiting room for hours with the other two. I could hear her screaming through two sets of closed doors, and they told me they were giving her all the medicine they dared. Doc, I get sick to my stomach when I hear her scream and realize I got her pregnant."

After receiving a "blue-edged guarantee" that he could leave any time he saw or heard anything that upset him—it being a free country—he reluctantly took the course. As he told us later he simply didn't believe a word of natural childbirth, he came only because his wife goaded him into it.

His wife was an intelligent, earnest woman who I just knew would be a good obstetrical athlete, and she was. During first-stage labor he sat fidgeting on the edge of his chair and looked so much like a little boy waiting for his first piano recital that his wife giggled. With gentle coaching she performed beautifully in the labor room, and, under the circumstances, so did he.

When the cervix was nearly dilated I suggested now that he accompany his wife to the delivery room for the actual birth. He panicked completely. He could still hear those screams from the other time. His wife said "Oh, come on, this is different," but he still held out. As the nurse took the calm mother to the delivery room I took the panic-stricken husband through the two sets of doors to the waiting room. On the way I had him help me prop the doors open, both sets. Then as he sat shakily in the waiting room I asked him when his wife began screaming to feel free to get up and close the doors. However, in case he didn't hear any screams he was still cordially invited to join his wife if he wished. Fortunately there were no other births going on that night. His wife was magnificent. We chatted between pushes. She kept giggling over her husband's fears.

He heard the chatter and giggles from his distant waiting room, but no screams. Finally loneliness and curiosity got the best of him and he came carefully around the corner, unfortunately just at the moment she was pushing hard with a contraction. As he saw her contorted red face (effort!) he panicked the second time, ran up to her and begged, "Take the gas, honey! Take the gas!"

She stopped pushing long enough to say, "Oh, get away, I'm busy!" Then in a few seconds she finished her push, looked up at his distraught face, and saved the whole situation by laughing uproariously at how *he* looked. This chagrined, but finally convinced, honest Dutchman became one of those so-called (by opponents) fanatics for the benefits of natural childbirth. I'm sure he would resent being called fanatical, because he could see and hear the difference between a medicated maniac and the same beloved woman as a calm, trained athlete who could interrupt her work just to kid him. It is significant how often these so-called fanatics for natural childbirth are people who have experienced medicated untrained childbirth first. Why aren't they fanatics for medicated deliveries?

Don't confuse the facial appearance of effort with that of pain. The more pressure your wife applies to her bottom, the better she feels and the better the baby will cry and expand its lungs at birth. This rhythmical intermittent mother pressure was meant to be, for both mother and baby.

Again let me throw in the challenge of testing the principles of the method. After you have satisfactorily coached your wife to take three big breaths, hold the third, squat, and try to move her bowels, ask her to not do any one of the three—see if there is a difference! Don't *believe* natural childbirth, *try* it.

Pressure on human flesh makes that area devoid of pain sensation—in proportion to the amount applied. You will find your wife earnestly pushing hard—for the simple reason that the harder she pushes, the better she feels. Why? Because pain perception is dependent upon circulating blood to the involved area, and pressure slows down or stops the circulation momentarily. This is really nothing new. The next time you see someone whack his shin accidentally on some object, watch what he does. He doesn't just look at his shin and say "Oh, fudge!" but will grab the shin and hold it in a tight grasp until it feels better.

The oldest anesthetic known to the battle surgeon was a tourniquet. Many a leg has been amputated painlessly without any anesthetic other than a properly applied tourniquet to stop circulation to the area involved. This occurs not only on the battlefield. There was a news article not too long ago about a forgetful but clever (I thought) intern who made an emergency run in an ambulance but forgot to take along his instruments (this is not apparently limited to plumbers). A man had had his leg mashed in an elevator accident and needed an immediate amputation. The intern borrowed a policeman's belt and club and applied an improvised tourniquet. With only this anesthetic he amputated the limb (probably with a borrowed knife!), for which the victim calmly thanked him.

Husbands sit on their "daddy stools" at the head end of the delivery room table and the doctor on "doctor stools" at the foot end. Many a time I have called up to the patient to stop cheating by letting air out her nose. One husband asked in bewilderment how I knew what her nose was doing when I was watching the other end. I couldn't see her nose from my view. The answer is really quite simple: while she was properly pushing, the area around her vagina blanched white from the pressure. When she let air out her nose the pressure was momentarily lessened and the circulation returned to this area which turned red. This didn't feel good and she would hold her breath again. I told her husband her bottom looked like a signal light blinking white and red, which informed me what she was doing. She laughed and pushed steadily instead of intermittently from then on.

Birth

As an observer you will notice that the time interval between contractions, which shortened to practically nothing in the crescendo or transition stage, now, in second stage, lengthens out again. The rest period becomes longer between contractions when the mother is called upon to work actively with her uterus. This is a very nice arrangement, as it gives the mother time to catch her breath and her self-control, enabling her to push more effectively. It also brings back a return of her communicability. Whereas in transition stage she became nonverbal as she concentrated on her work, in second stage she may resume her talking between contractions; there's time enough now. Recalling the mountain climbing comparison, you two are now traversing the more gradual plateau that leads to the summit and there is time for pleasantries. She may ask you to perform little tasks (wiping her brow with a cold cloth, moistening her lips, adjusting the pillows more to her satisfaction, etc.). During the pushing stage we suggest that you no longer give her ice chips as you did in the labor room. If she complains of dryness of her lips let her bite down on the cold moist cloth you have. The attending nurse can give you some mineral oil or vaseline to lubricate her lips occasionally. Like an athlete engaged in the most strenuous part of the performance, she should keep her stomach empty now until the job is done. If she fills it with anything at this stage, the stomach will reject it. Keep it empty but reassure her that she will soon be finished and she can have her iced orange juice shortly, when the job is completed. The swimmer waits until he has finished the long swim before he eats or drinks. Following these simple rules, we have had no trouble with upset stomachs. Any mother can eat a full meal after the orange juice.

As the baby begins to "crown," that is, stretch the external vaginal lips until they surround its head like a crown, your wife may exhibit a change in her reactions to what's going on. She now knows by the way it feels (the external skin is more sensitive to feeling) that the baby is actually coming out and that the long awaited moment is here. Women act differently at this moment. It is an exciting, provocative feeling. I think it is best described, and the emotions that accompany it, by Helen Wessel who speaks of the "birth climax" and compares the high emotional content favorably with the sensations a woman feels in reaching a full sexual orgasm with the man she loves. Your wife may, as she feels the baby coming out, give a little squeal of ecstasy. She may cry out in surprise over the momentary new sensation of the baby passing through the external lips. This is probably related to the fact that the clitoris, which is the sensitive passion center point at the front of the vagina, where the minor lips come together and surround it, is now being stimulated by the passage of the baby, giving a definite sensual feeling to this moment. It is only a momentary fleeting feeling. Some women make no outcry at all (as is true in sexual orgasms). It is attended with great emotional feeling either way. I have observed mothers spontaneously wrapping their arms around their husband's neck, kissing, crying with joy, squealing with delight, etc. I always feel like an intruder and outsider to an intimate relationship between man and wife. I would feel embarrassed if the husband weren't there!

Mrs. Wessel's term "birth climax" fits the very frank answers to our queries of unmedicated mothers whose husbands were with them. We have had this comparison with a love climax brought up before.

One mother gave us a very complete description of the sensations of birth. The bowel movement comparison was during the gradual descent of the baby as it traversed the internal vaginal canal. The rectum is located between the descending baby's head and the forward curving lower portion of the backbone (sacrum). Although the rectum is empty, the pressure from the downward sliding baby is manifested against the rectum, due to the unyielding nature of the backbone behind it and the physical phenomenon of going around a curve. We refer to the lovely curve of the derrière of ladies as the baby sliding board. It is very similar to those playground sliding boards in schoolyards as it curves forward and upward in the lower half, and both were made for children to traverse.

In descending, the baby, after it has gone around the curve of the sacrum, comes forward as it actually leaves the mother's body and places tension and pressure—for the first time and only momentarily, at the actual moment of passage—in the clitoral region. In a love climax this is the area that receives and gives vigorous pressure as part of the ecstasy experience. At the moment our patient's baby was born her husband told her afterward that she made sounds just as she did in a love climax.

Could this experience between two people who love each other combined with the thrilling privilege of seeing for the first time the product of their blended love—their baby—be related to the nuisance they make ever after to be together when subsequent babies are to be born? Experienced natural childbirth parents are never nonchalant in their desire to share this event. Husbands have been known to leave no stones unturned in their determination to be with their wives—e.g., the college student who chained himself to his wife in labor because "I love her," the legally oriented ones who have applied injunctions and legal restraints over their physical exclusion from delivery rooms, and others of like nature.

One of our highly intelligent husbands, Terence Cory, a newswriter for ABC-TV, was not a natural childbirth "fanatic" with the first two children. He was an excellent father and labor coach, very happy and satisfied with the good show his wife Ginny put on under his direction. He was not a fanatic for natural childbirth—that is, not until he had moved to Chicago and his wife became pregnant again. He found out, to his fury, that the state of Illinois still had backward, old laws (purposeful in the "knock 'em out, drag 'em out" era) which ignored and defeated all principles of family-centered childbirth. He became a fanatic in a very short time. A man of action and connected with the TV industry, he decided his contribution would be to have a public debate on TV between professional people advocating natural childbirth with husbands as active participants, and those professional people who were against these concepts. I warned him that those against would decline an open debate, as the public is on the other side and it's an uncomfortable position to assume. However he was determined to try. Try he did, but the show went on with only those advocating the principles present; the others declined. Their negative part was voiced by the interviewer and cut to ribbons by the enthusiastic advocates.

In 1947 I first experimented with these concepts and ran up against opposition from nearly all angles—medical, hospital administrative, nursing supervisors, etc. I made a prediction then that, troublesome as may be the necessary changes in obstetrical management inherent in natural childbirth, we were dealing not with minor techniques of management but with major human rights, human rights which seem superficially simple and obvious —the right of a woman to bear her children with all her mental faculties and her husband present, if she wishes. Whether the medical profession liked these concepts or not, they would have them jammed down their reluctant throats by public demand. This was met with laughter then. The laughter has faded now.

We have had patients fly to Denver from California in order to have babies with their husbands participating. While I'm writing, a legal test is going on in California by a handful of "medical Daniels" who dare to be different. They are backed by an ever growing group of lay, legal, and medical people who know their rights and are determined, in a free country, that they shall have them. In Madison, Wisconsin, mothers are sticking their tongues out impudently at rigid hospital rules and driving to Milwaukee in labor where rules have been changed.

However, the following quote from the *AMA News* of January 1, 1965 indicates that young husbands and fathers-to-be should give a thought to possible consequences before they invade delivery rooms.

DELIVERY ROOM 'INVADER' FINED

A New Jersey father who gained unauthorized admission to a hospital's delivery room in an attempt to witness the birth of his second child last July was told by a Union, N.J., County Court judge in November that the incident will cost the father $150.

Judge Ervin S. Fulop upheld a conviction and fine by Plainfield Municipal Court Magistrate Warren J. Lynch last August against John O. Keim, 33, on charges that he acted in a disorderly manner when he refused to leave his wife's side in the delivery room at Plainfield's Muhlenberg Hospital on July 17. In appealing, Keim contended that he had caused no trouble and that he did not know three men, summoned to the delivery room to ask him to leave, were policemen.

A hospital nurse had told the Municipal Court that she notified Keim that layman fathers were not permitted into the delivery room under hospital regulations, but only into the labor room. Mrs. Iris Keim was moved quickly to the delivery room after her arrival at the hospital. The nurse said that Keim's insistence on going into the delivery room led her to give him surgical garb while permission was asked for him to be admitted.

When the request was denied and Keim entered anyway, just moments after his daughter had been born, the nurse phoned the police. Three policemen wearing surgical clothing went in the delivery room, but Keim reportedly still would not leave. He told the court that an earlier pregnancy of his wife ended in a miscarriage, that his wife had German measles during the recent pregnancy, and that she was two weeks late in delivering this child.

Now, back to the birth room and your role as a coach. After the final push, accompanied by surprised squeals of delight, get your heads together. Put your head down with your wife's, cheek to cheek. Hold her hand under the sterile sheet—she's through pushing with it, grasp her hand, love her, praise her, share her joy. Actually, I don't need to direct you to do this. If you're there you just can't help but share her joy; it is contagious to all present but particularly to the one who loves her. I have seen tears of shared joy unashamedly in the eyes of husbands at this moment. Do remember not to touch the top of the sheet, either of you—rules, you know!

After the baby is born there will be a slight lull during which the doctor holds the baby upside down by grasping the child's ankles. This lull is during the time the salt water (amniotic fluid) is running from the baby's lungs. All babies' lungs are filled with amniotic fluid in the uterus. As soon as the water runs out you two will hear the sweetest sound on earth, the first cry of your baby. In unmedicated births it is hardly ever necessary for the doctor to spank the baby; he merely holds it upside down and wipes it clean with gauze squares.

When I first practiced husband participation, I inadvertently frightened the alert observant parents by not having prepared them for the fact that we always hold the baby down lower than the mother's abdomen, as well as upside down, immediately at birth. They thought I was deliberately hiding the baby from their view and looked fearfully at each other ("Why won't he let us see the baby? Is there something wrong with it?").

Natural childbirth with the husband's participation is definitely a nuisance to doctors. If the mother were asleep and the father out pacing the waiting room, there would be no need for books or prenatal classes to explain carefully in advance every little detail of what we do and, because of the intelligence of our patients, *why* we do it. One of the hazards of this method in the eyes of medical opponents is the fact that both parents are allowed to see their baby at birth, even if something is wrong with it—an exceedingly rare occurrence. I do not personally deem this a hazard, as there is no point in misleading parents into thinking their baby is all right, then shocking them with the truth at some later time. This would be far more upsetting than being told or shown the truth in the first place. Honesty is still the best policy in all human dealings.

We do not "hide" babies from parents. Why, then, do we hold the baby so low that you can't see it, immediately after it is born? To allow gravity action to siphon baby blood back out of the placenta—which at this moment is still in the mother's uterus. The baby wants back the blood he has donated to the placenta, and immediately at birth the umbilical cord is open and serves as a hose through which the blood can flow from the placenta back into the baby. If we put the baby immediately up on top of the mother's abdomen so that you can see it, the baby's blood would tend by gravity action to leave the baby and flow into the placenta. Some opponents of natural childbirth get the mistaken idea—possibly from the action in the French movie *The Case of Dr. Laurent*—that we show the baby in this position immediately after birth just to cater to the parents. The movie version was, I hope, a slip-up in a staged drama and has no basis in fact. Natural childbirth does not ever depart from any obstetrical principles; it adds, but never subtracts.

The doctor, then, will hold your baby down as low as the umbilical cord will allow until he is satisfied that the blood has ceased flowing back into the baby. He can tell this by the appearance of narrowing and whitening of the cord or by feeling it with his fingers as you would feel a hose to see if there is liquid running in it. This only takes a minute or two, and when it is completed he will then hand your baby to your wife, cord still intact, to hold through the sterile sheet or drape that is over her abdomen.

How anyone after a moment's reflection on animal births would think that in imitating animals in the management of human births we would place the baby higher than the placenta is inconceivable to me. After all, animal babies are always lower than their mother's abdomen at birth!

As a husband, keep your seat on your daddy stool at all times. Do not get up and wander around to get a preliminary view. You would get in the way of the attendants and disrupt the normal procedures. Wait to share your wife's view of the baby. She should not try to be a contortionist and peer over her abdomen. Be patient a few minutes. You will hear your baby cry before you will see it. Take joy in the sound. Praise your wife for her good performance, keep your head next to hers, and share the view together.

During the few moments while the doctor is holding the baby low many things are happening. Your doctor will use a rubber bulb syringe to suck the mucous and salt water out of your baby's nose and mouth—he hasn't learned to spit or blow his nose as yet; you can teach him that later. The doctor will also be tilting the baby's head backward to let gravity assist in draining the nose, sinuses, and mouth. He will take gauze squares and be wiping the baby clean—or cleaner—during this time. Internally, miracles are happening. Valves are automatically closing in the umbilicus to prevent baby blood from running back in the cord. Valves are closing in the baby's heart, valves that remained open during the intrauterine life to direct blood through the cord and placenta to pick up oxygen and nourishment from the mother via the placental surface. Other valves that remained closed are now opening for the first time, allowing the blood that used to go to the placenta for oxygen to circulate now through the baby's lungs, which now contain air for the first time. Isn't it a miracle that these parts know how to do these things at the proper time?

Now the baby is ready to be handed to your wife to hold through the sheet. Neither you nor your wife should touch it directly. Both of you will tend by reflex to want to touch and feel the baby—don't. Not yet. You will have plenty of time for that later. Your wife can hold the baby to her breast by handling it through the sheet covering her abdomen. If later on the baby is going to be placed in a nursery, even temporarily, with other babies, bacteria from your hands may spread in the nursery to other babies. Even if your hospital is modern and has rooming-in arrangements, the baby may be removed temporarily to the nursery during night hours. It is best to wait until the baby is home; then you can handle it all you wish.

If you have never seen a newborn baby before, I think it would be beneficial to know in advance what to expect. It is a pinky-purple hue at birth. The blue element comes from the normal fact that it has extra blood at birth, more than it really needs. This is a leftover from the intrauterine life where the extra blood was necessary, as it got its oxygen secondhand from its mother's blood. This extra blood will gradually be disposed of, which gives the baby a yellowish or jaundiced color about its third day of life. At the moment of birth it imparts a bluish tint which when combined with the red color of a healthy baby gives a pinky-purple result.

Also when babies are just born there is a layer of built-in fat just under the skin together with a normal state of puffiness of the skin (edema) which gives the baby's face a jowly, ponderous look. One mother told her husband all her newborn babies looked just the way he did in the mornings after a big party.

The baby has been in darkness for nine months and the sudden introduction to light makes him squint. Another mother said newborn babies looked to her like Mr. Magoo, the nearsighted squinting cartoon character. After a period of adjustment of about five to ten minutes the baby will open his eyes. Do not expect some preconceived color of your baby's eyes at birth—they are all gray-blue and achieve adult colors later.

The baby's head will appear elongated and perhaps just a little lopsided. Don't worry about it; it's supposed to look like that due to the "molding" effect of its position in the birth canal. There may be a little puffy area of the scalp, usually to one side of the dome, which is called the "cap of birth" and comes from the gradual dilatation of the cervix. All these little irregularities will gradually fade out in a few days and are normal.

Newborn babies' skin will be wet with salt water and have irregular blotches of grayish yellow material here and there, which we dub "baby cold cream." It is actually accumulated skin oil and has the impressive name *vernix caseosa.* In ancient times it was thought to have magical properties and was carefully saved and used for multiple purposes, medical and otherwise. One use was to rub on gun stocks as special wood preservative by gun collectors.

Do not jump to conclusions about the color or consistency of the baby's hair. It is wet with salt water and may appear curly when it actually isn't. We refer to newborn babies' hair as "puppy fuzz" because it is so fine and, as with puppies, the color at birth may change somewhat later.

If the doctor has done an episiotomy while your wife was pushing—and no anesthetic other than pressure and whiteness of the flesh being cut is necessary—he will inject novocaine in the edges of the cut and put in the necessary few stitches while you and your wife are counting fingers and toes and playing with the baby. He will then tie or clamp the umbilical cord.

If your wife is going to breast-feed, the doctor will ask the nurse to help your wife put the baby to the breast right on the delivery room table. The nurse will cleanse the nipple with an antiseptic solution and help place the baby in the hollow of the mother's arm, working again through the sheet that is over the abdomen.

The baby will not be particularly interested in eating—he has built-in nourishment for about three days—but he will like the warmth of your wife's breast and will receive a sticky substance called colostrum from it. The main beneficiary of the maneuver will be your wife. The uterus contracts by reflex from breast stimulation, which also helps to separate the placenta from its contact with the uterus. It further helps to reduce the size of the uterus to nonpregnant proportions, and by contracting serves to shut off the maternal blood vessels which formerly fed the baby.

Your wife will feel the placenta slip out of the uterus and down against her vagina, from five to ten minutes after the birth.

Many doctors assist the placenta in coming out in different ways. Some push on the abdomen, some ask the mother to bear down and expel it, or some gently tug on the cord—or combinations of all three.

The passage of the placenta is called the third stage of labor. Animals instinctively eat their placentas after they are passed. The animal mothers chew the cord in two, at a safe long distance from the baby. They then give little pulls on the cord until the placenta is passed. We similarly give little tugs on the cord to see if the placenta has separated. If it hasn't we wait a few moments and tug again. When it has separated from the uterus your wife will feel a full feeling in her vagina followed by a delightfully empty feeling, as the doctor lifts the placenta out by traction on the cord. Her big tummy is now fully emptied of the baby, the water, and the "baby house," or placenta. We usually hear admiring comments from both husband and wife as they compare the size of abdomen now with the size it was a few minutes before.

If you want to see a placenta and your doctor has the time after you are all through, have him wash it off and show it to you.

It is a magical organ that contains many undiscovered secrets of function and of secretions. The reason animals eat theirs is probably related to some substance it contains which serves to stimulate uterine contractions. Your doctor may give you an injection of an oxytocic drug which serves the same purpose. In early days human placentas were said to have been dried, ground up, and compressed into pill form and fed mothers postpartum.

However, today we have many good chemicals which serve the same purpose. Let your doctor decide if, when, and whether your wife needs them. With our many enthusiastic breast-feeding mothers we do not always give an oxytocin; it depends on how well the uterus contracts. This varies with every mother and every pregnancy.

After the baby, placenta, and episiotomy stitches, if any, are completed the mother should be given the iced orange juice to restore her depleted blood sugar that was used up by the uterine muscle action during the course of labor. It is, as we have mentioned, also refreshing to the mouth, which has become quite dry from mouth breathing. In the spirit of sharing childbirth we also offer the father a glass of iced orange juice with his wife as a little token of doctor gratitude—share and share alike.

Shortly after the baby is born and placenta expelled your wife may experience a mild shaky chilly sensation. This is not due to coldness or to nervousness as some mothers immediately assume. Rather it is due to the physiological changes in circulation incident to the now empty uterus. It is only a momentary phenomenon and is normal.

At this happy moment in two people's lives (or should it be three?) we teasingly state in a dry matter-of-fact voice that "Next time we'll keep the husband away, put the mother to sleep, and *deliver* the baby ourself." The opponents of natural childbirth should hear the assortment of return comments that invokes! Its prime purpose is to trigger grateful sincere statements from the wife directed to the husband: "Honey, I don't know what I'd have done without you."

Walking back from the birth room has become associated with natural childbirth since its earliest inception. It is not necessary, and if the mother labored during usual sleep hours we do not advise it. (Of course if she has had medication or complications it is out of the question.) However, we have had thousands of mothers who insist on walking back and quite frankly take delight in doing so. The other day, in the wee small hours of morning, one of our repeater mothers gave birth, and because of the hour I suggested she ride back to her room. She saucily stuck her tongue out at me and walked out of the room with her beaming husband.

I find it hard to argue with these obstetrical athletes. It's equally hard to find them as I make hospital rounds—they simply don't stay in bed; they keep insisting they are not sick, so why should they stay in bed?

Any young doctor who devotes a little time and energy to setting up a training course in natural childbirth, I give fair warning, will be resented by his colleagues as a patient stealer. Most hospitals have recovery rooms on obstetrical floors where all patients are taken for a two-hour period after they have babies. The exuberant natural childbirth mothers look so good, feel so good, and act so happy that the medicated or anesthetic-recovering ones ask them how come. In that two-hour stay with several other patients in the same room, believe me, they find out how come. Having once experienced natural childbirth, the parents, I have noticed, are never reluctant to talk about it.

The greatest handicap we have found in practicing natural childbirth has always been the overenthusiasm of our patients. Of course it's a two-edged sword, and if medicated patients looked, felt, and acted better than nonmedicated ones, the promotion would be for the other side.

6

The Coach's Training Rules

COACHES do not function only during the game. They are essential in the physical preparation of the *body* during the training course long before the game. They should also prepare the athlete's *mind* so that there is a clear conception and understanding of the duties involved. They should by their interest and enthusiasm be a living symbol to the *spirit* of the player, motivating the individual to want to play the game at his level best.

The same applies to your duties as a husband and coach to prepare your obstetrical athlete properly for the great event—labor and the birth of your child.

Why bother? Why let all this new rigmarole possibly interfere with your golf game? Women have babies, that's their job.

Buster, you have to live with this baby factory. If your act of love results in the changing of your wife from a pretty, stimulating companion, a warm, affectionate, passionate lover, and a charmer who "likes being a girl"—to a sway-backed, varicose-veined, round-shouldered slob; to a cold, frigid ("Get away from me") rejecter of affection, to a hostile resenter of a woman's role ("Men have it easy!"), you have no one to blame but yourself. If you think this is an exaggeration compare a few of your older friends' wives with what they used to look like, act like, and feel like before they had babies.

Parents come in pairs. If you think the only task you have as a parent is to get your wife pregnant, you're going to be like the farmer who thinks all there is to farming is planting seeds. You will harvest only the weeds of resentment to your passivity. You are poorly prepared for parenthood and have yet to recognize your responsibilities. Your schooling didn't prepare you—they teach typing, tap dancing, and tomfoolery but precious little preparation for parenthood. Your parents probably didn't prepare you. No one ever prepared them—they cannot pass on to you what they didn't receive. The rising divorce rate reflects what pitiful examples of parenthood many couples are.

Maybe I'm old-fashioned and in this complex modern society serial polygamy is the answer. Don't kid yourself, the hand that rocks the cradle still rules the world, and always will. Motherly women and fatherly men acting as wholesome symbols of strength and righteousness in a family setting of mutual love and respect continue to be essential to progress in any civilization.

It is true that the methods of achieving this ideal state change somewhat with changing times. I doubt very much if your grandparents and possibly your parents will be in full agreement with all the concepts set forth in this book. But then, women are not chained to the kitchen any more; they even join the men in the library after dinner to discuss politics—they too can vote!

The reaction your wife has to her pregnancy and the birth of *your* child will reflect on the relationship between you as man and wife, and it will reflect on the relationship between mother and child forever after. Will she look upon childbearing as a horrifying ordeal that ruined her figure and seared her soul? Will she awaken from an anesthetic with a curse on her lips—"Never again; *you* have the next one"?

Or will she joyfully share with you even the little nuisances involved and thank you for getting her pregnant, and bless her God for the privilege of being a woman and of giving birth. I recall one trained young mother who squealed in delight at the moment of birth, "that was fun!" Then she added as she ecstatically kissed her husband, "Oh, honey, when can we have another one?"

I hadn't had time to dry off this baby and she was looking forward already to the next. These are the mothers with active participating husbands whose understanding, encouragement, and guidance of their wives constitute the most important factors in natural childbirth.

You are going to live with this woman until "death do us part." How rich, full, and meaningful that life will be is very much dependent upon your ability as a participant in parenthood. This does not exclude but takes precedence over the golf game, pool hall, poker game, etc.

Let's get on with it. What are your responsibilities as a coach:

Physical Conditioning

I'm sure you have had similar experiences but let me use one of mine to illustrate a point. I had been away from the old home town for eight years attending school. On a nostalgic return to visit relatives and old friends I happened to meet the girl who had been judged the prettiest in our high school class. I had to be told who she was, and even then found it hard to believe. I remembered her as a statuesquely beautiful, poised "sweater girl," whose sparkling eyes reflected the joy of living. I now saw before me a sway-backed, round-shouldered, sagging, varicose-veined slouch whose dull, listless face reflected the boredom of life. I exclaimed in amazement to a friend, "What happened to her?" His answer: "Oh, she's had several babies since you last saw her and they just ruined her figure." I take vigorous exception to this statement. No baby ever ruined any woman's figure; mothers ruin their own figures! Don't keep blaming the innocent babies.

Now, unfortunately, you can't in all honesty blame the woman entirely. One must blame society and ignorance. Having babies need not ruin a mother's figure.

There are thousands of statuesquely beautiful natural childbirth mothers whose bodies remain beautiful after many babies. Our three R.N. exercise teachers, having had three babies apiece, attest to this fact. They serve not only as teachers but as shining examples. On an invited lecture tour in Ottawa, Canada, I had the pleasure of sitting with Dick Hartman, the young husband of one (a Canadian R.N.). We both beamed with pride watching his leotard-clad wife, Rhondda, on a TV program as she demonstrated the adaptation of housework and baby care to the beneficial "mother-like" way of doing things. Her slim body and good posture spoke more than words, and she had had two babies and was in early pregnancy with her third! There are some things your wife can do and some ways of doing those things which as a mother she must do that will preserve physical beauty. These things do not necessarily fit Emily Post's way of being "ladylike" but rather the natural childbirth concept of being "mother-like."

PRENATAL EXERCISES:

The term "exercises" tends to immediately tire some women by its very connotation. I would prefer to call them "body mechanisms of pregnancy." Most of them are simply ways of doing what any housewife and/or mother must do anyway. Our fervent plea is, do it! Now here is where we have depended totally on husbands' cooperation as "pregnancy policemen." Your wife really means to follow directions at all times, but Emily Post's suggestions of how to act ladylike have been established for years as a habit pattern. We have found by careful follow-up that what your wife means to do and what she does may be two totally different acts. She needs to be constantly reminded to act mother-like in the privacy of her home.

It is not the intention of this book to teach your wife *how* to do the necessary exercises, rather to teach you as a husband *why* you should see to it that she does them.

Your wife can learn them in two ways—by going to natural childbirth exercise classes, where they are demonstrated and performed, or by studying a text. The first is, of course, far preferable, but if no classes are available in your locality, don't give up. Write the headquarters of the I.C.E.A. and ask for information. If you still find there are no classes within a reasonable distance of where you live, the exercises can be learned from a book. They are clearly set forth in *Natural Childbirth and the Christian Family* by Helen Wessel; *Childbirth Without Fear* by Dr. Grantly Dick-Read, and *Relaxation and Exercises for Natural Childbirth* by Helen Heardman. The first two are published by Harper & Row, the third by Williams and Wilkins.

The motivation in wanting your wife to actually participate in exercise classes is twofold. First I think the exercises are easier for her to learn by observing the teacher doing them and then having the teacher observe her doing them. The second motivation is that although we label these classes "physical training" for natural childbirth, actually one cannot completely divorce the body from the mind. There is a great psychological benefit from association with experienced natural childbirth mothers. (You and I, husband and doctor, can talk until we're blue in the face but glib as we may be there is a great handicap: we're men and we've never *had* a baby.) We deliberately mix experienced natural childbirth mothers into these classes and thereby create a setup for a female gab session—a hen party where your wife can verbalize with birds of like feather.

Let's assume your wife knows how to do these exercises from either classes or books. Now, as a man, you will want to know enough about them so that you can tell if your wife is doing them properly, and, most important, *why* they must be done. What is the logic and reasoning behind them? Nothing gets done if it doesn't appear reasonable, and very frankly if your wife went to class, learned the exercises, and came home and performed, you might feel the urge to call the paddy wagon to come and get her. The exercises look idiotic, some of them. They are not idiotic, they just look that way. Why? Because of the unhandy location of the baby box on a woman. Why it was put in this particular location, God only knows, literally. A zippered "baby door" on your wife's abdomen would have been far handier, but we must learn to take things the way they come!

Let's not lose sight of the coming event—labor and birth—as an athletic event. It is this in a very true sense. Let's repeat again, it's darned hard work and the term *labor* is most appropriate. The amount of energy involved is comparable to that a football player uses playing a full game of football, every minute, with no substitution.

A player who entered such a game without having had any recent experience or taken any special training to condition the muscles involved would be so stiff and sore and miserable after the game was over that he probably would have to be carried from the field.

Similarly, a mother, given nine months' notice of game time, who makes no physical preparation yet when the whistle blows must play the full game (there is no substitution here) would have to be carried from the field and would do well if she could walk comfortably within several days thereafter.

Conversely, an athlete who takes cognizance of the physical conditioning of the muscles involved and performs daily training exercises during these preliminary months to get in condition has no trouble walking off the field when the game is over. A physically prepared natural childbirth mother often makes a nuisance of herself (to hospital attendants, that is) by walking back from the birth room.

The muscles involved in your obstetrical athlete are the three B's—back, belly, and bottom. These are the ones which must be strengthened and made flexible, and have the stiffness of disuse worked out of them by daily calisthenics—just as for any other athlete.

Most prenatal exercise classes exclude the husband because of the unhandy location of the obstetrical muscles. Don't let this hurt your male ego that you're not invited. It's just that it's a bit awkward for your wife to learn to tighten and loosen her vaginal muscles, attired in unladylike garments, in front of other women's husbands. (Our patients wear leotards or similar garments at exercise classes.) Some of the exercises your wife will be taught you cannot help her with or coach her in—e.g., the perineal, pubococcygeal, or "Kegel" one. However, there are other important ones where she will need your help and your reminding.

Let's begin with the ones which do not represent any expenditure of extra time on her part, but rather are simply mother-like ways of doing what she's going to be doing anyway.

1. *Sitting.* This could hardly be called an exercise, as it represents an inactivity, yet it can be done in such a way that it will stretch and make flexible the muscles on her bottom and the inner aspects of her thighs that will allow her to put her legs farther apart in second-stage labor—or open the baby door wider when the time comes.

This approved and appropriate way for her to sit is most unladylike and she can't do it in public. But she can jolly well do it in private, and it's your job to see that she does!

It is called "tailor sitting" or "Indian style," or "kid sitting," or in Yogi circles the "lotus position." It should preferably be done on a hard surface like the floor so the crossed feet will be on the same level as the hips. Your wife should lean forward and put her elbows on her knees and her work (sewing, writing, snapping green beans, etc.) on the floor before her. This serves to let her enlarging uterus fall freely forward (where it belongs!) instead of tipping backward (where it doesn't belong). The leaning forward bends the bow (her back) and thereby loosens the bowstring (her abdominal muscles), thus allowing the uterus room to come forward.

The principles behind this position of sitting can be illustrated in many ways. First, it's the most comfortable way there is to sit. Let any child alone and he will not sit in a chair; with his legs together, and if you turn your back he won't stay there long, you'll find. Obstinate brat? No, it's uncomfortable. Kids are far more comfortable sitting on the floor—reading the funny papers or books, etc. If left alone they will continue to do this auto-matically even up to teen age.

Tailors have sat that way since time immemorial for the simple reason they sit all the time in their work and found this position the most comfortable way there is to sit.

It is a "natural" way to sit, as manifested in American Indians, Africans, Chinese, Japanese—the entire Orient and much of the rest of the world.

Among these peoples varicose veins of the legs, hemorrhoids, uterine prolapses (fallen wombs), etc., occur far less often than they do in Westernized countries where people are forced by custom to sit in chairs. This is not the only factor involved, of course but it is an important one.

Sitting erect in a chair or, even worse, slumped backwards in a chair will make your wife's uterus descent deeply into the pelvis instead of freely falling forward. It compresses the large blood vessels going to the kidneys and legs and interferes with circulation to these parts.

Then adding insult to injury, someone long ago decreed that ladies do not sit with their legs apart. That it is ladylike to cross their legs! Ah, brother, we do have problems with your wife. (See cartoon ℞ Modesty, from "Medical Directors Notebook".)

I have jokingly told my classes that I'm tempted to move to Russia after reading an article in the newspaper the other day about an English girl who caused a traffic jam in Moscow because she was wearing heavy red stockings. It seemed that this color is the advertising sign of a prostitute in Russia! The article went on about the different customs and described how Russian women never cross their legs in public, as they consider this vulgar! Would God we could borrow *their* etiquette director for a while! Leg-crossing further cuts off circulation to the legs and to the vagina itself.

You and I are not asking your wife to assume a Russian sprawl in public but, rather, giving voice to the first great command-ment for pregnant women: Thou shalt not sit in a chair in private. It is your job as her companion in privacy to see to it that this commandment is obeyed. Those legs were pretty when you married her, see that you keep them that way! She is going to have occasion to sit at home, so just be sure she sits the approved way. Now she mustn't be forced to sit in *any* position, including our approved one, for great lengths of time. Long periods of

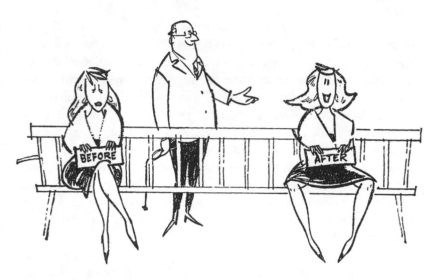

inactivity also make for poor circulation and stiff muscles. Rather she should putter around. If any of her housework such as peeling potatoes or polishing silver, normally performed standing up or sitting in a chair, can be done sitting on the floor tailor-fashion, this is ideal, but no position should be maintained for too long. Pregnant women should also eat meals off the coffee table while sitting on the floor as often as possible.

In the later months of pregnancy, when her uterus is quite large, it is permissible, for short periods of time, for her to sit contour-chair style with her legs sprawled comfortably apart and elevated higher than her hips.

Ordinary lawn chairs of contour variety serve well for this purpose, or using pillows or blankets to lend appropriate support on the divan is permissible. The uterus is so large it tends to fall forward from its own weight, even in this semisitting position. Variety in position also serves to make a break in the monotony.

It should be obvious that your wife should wear flexible or loose-fitting garments that allow complete freedom of movement.

2. *Squatting.* Your wife will have many occasions to get down to do something in her household duties. If you have no children as yet, this would be in getting a pan out of the lower shelf in the kitchen, picking up around the house (your socks?), polishing the floor, etc. I once checked on a housewife without children to see how many occasions she had to "get down" in the course of one day—it was about twenty-five. I then observed a young mother with small children and it was over a hundred times!

Here is the magnificent opportunity for your wife to prepare the muscles in all three B's—back, belly, and bottom—while performing her chores. Squatting is, again, unladylike, especially the way the exercise teacher will show your wife to rise from this position—tail first!

Again, you don't have to attend a special class to have this simple natural way of doing something (getting down and back up) demonstrated. Just watch a small child at play. The little girl toddler will comfortably squat for long periods (it's a natural position) while playing with her dolls, or jacks, or what have you. (So did your wife when she was that age and her squatting muscles didn't protest one bit.) When the little toddler rises she comes up from the squat "tail first" and then straightens all the way up. So did your wife at that age, and pregnancy commandment number two is—so shall she now! Coach's training rules!

If you observe your wife in the privacy of your home keeping her legs locked straight and bending her back—jamming her pregnant uterus deeper in the pelvis, misusing her lower back muscles that alone must support the pelvic contents—smite her gently but firmly on the most prominent portion of her anatomy (her buttocks) and remind her to put same down against her heels where it belongs.

Why? There's that question again. Experience has shown that the noninstinctive but ever-so-reasoning human animal always performs better if he knows why.

Many reasons why. The first in importance is that this squatting position is the very position that your wife must assume at the actual birth of her baby. If her muscles are so stiff from disuse and unfamiliarity with this position that she cannot properly assume it, may God have mercy on her bottom and her baby! It is the physical means of opening the baby door to let the baby out. The farther apart her knees can go, the farther back her thighs can go, the wider the door is opened, and the sooner and more comfortably the baby comes out.

The importance of the physical factor of legs apart to let a baby out was illustrated in a gruesome, negative way by an article in *Ladies Home Journal*, December 1958, titled "Cruelty in Maternity Wards." This consisted of a series of letters from indignant mothers justly criticizing their obstetrical care. The majority were in condemnation of the practice of nurses holding the mothers' legs together until the doctor got there. What happens if a mother cannot spread her legs apart when the baby is wanting to get out? First, of course, it can't get out. Second, nature punishes mothers who do the wrong thing—it hurts! Pain is purposeful: it's a sign of something wrong. No one can rightly argue with those mothers whose legs were held together. There is never justification for such treatment. In justice to the nurses involved it was not their fault—they act only upon doctor's orders. The third thing that was obvious in the many letters: it's not good for the baby to be held back.

We instruct our patients always that if they are ever caught inadvertently with a baby knocking at the baby door, wanting to get out, to squat and push the baby out. It matters not who is around or where they may be at the time. Policemen, mailmen, firemen, and Boy Scouts (both with and without a first-aid badge) have been known to "deliver" babies under emergency nonhospital situations, and two results stand out significantly as a consequence: (1) how well the mother gets along, and (2) how well the baby gets along.

Isn't that a silly word, "deliver"? Would it deflate the ego of the attendant at such a *birth* if it were pointed out that both mother and baby would have done fine if left alone?

Would it hurt their pride if it were pointed out that umbilical cords don't have to be cut and tied at all—that it's better just to leave them alone and intact?

Back to the legs-apart business. What if a woman through ignorance has never, since early childhood, sat with her legs apart? What if these muscles are so stiff from disuse that she can only put her legs halfway apart? If she can only open the door halfway it's going to take longer and hurt more than if she were capable of opening the baby door all the way. What if unfounded anxieties, resulting from negative conditioning for years, makes her afraid to spread her legs apart to let the baby out? She's afraid it will hurt to let the baby pass. No one ever convinced her in advance that the exact opposite is true: it hurts the mother *and* the baby if legs are not spread apart!

The squatting position is important. See that your wife is acquainted with it and gets more so as her pregnancy progresses.

No, your wife doesn't squat on the ground or floor at the moment of birth—although there is no good mechanical reason why she couldn't have a baby there, except it's a bit unhandy for the doctor and nurse, and floors aren't noted for being the cleanest of receptacles for newborn babies. (See cartoon.)[1]

We still use the delivery room table, but we also still use the squatting position on it. This is accomplished by tilting the table forward (they're adjustable) as far as is convenient and propping

[1] "All right, then, have it *your* way." from "Cartoon Classics," *Medical Economics, Inc.*

your wife's curved back up with pillows, or that most favorite of adjustable back supports, a knowledgable cooperating husband. (See Chapter 5)

In the historical development of the importance of the squatting position it was stressed by the late Helen Heardman, distin-

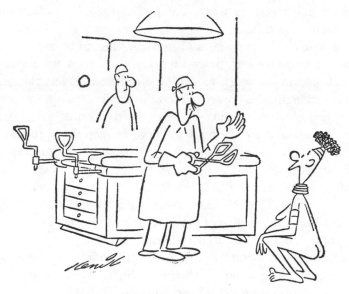

"All right, then, have it your way!"

guished English physiotherapist, that boat women in India who labored (employment) in the squatting position, pulling canal boats along, also labored (birth!) with ease to produce their young. It has also been described in other Oriental mothers as a contributing factor to the ease of birth. The paucity of varicose veins, hemorrhoids, uterine prolapses, and such among these peoples undoubtedly is related to the frequency of this position in their daily lives.

Members of all social strata in the Orient move their bowels in this position. Those in the lower social strata also work long hours, men and women alike, in the squatting position in the fields. At one of our informal prenatal meetings a husband interrupted to describe a scene he had oberved in China during World War II. He was riding as a passenger in a military convoy. He noted a woman worker interrupt her work momentarily, squat by the side of the field, give birth to a baby, place it in a sling on her back and return to work—completing the entire affair while the convoy was passing!

You wife need not go around squatting just to be squatting. It is merely a sensible way of getting down and back up when she has occasion in her work to do this, for instance, scrubbing the floor, working in the flower garden, loving, buttoning, or spanking young children. Again, she can take the pan of green beans from the sink and put them on the floor to snap them. Instead of that misery-producing half bend over the sink she can keep her back straight and bend her legs, squatting on the floor, to perform the same task. The Creator put hinges at the knees and hips, not on the back; encourage your wife to use these hinges. Straight backs and bent legs never harmed any pregnant woman. Straight legs and bent backs have harmed many.

Some pregnant women in the older age group will complain of a pulling or aching feeling in the inner thighs when first performing their squatting exercise. Especially so if it has been years and years since their bodies have assumed this position. This is not a sign that all is lost and they can't do what others do.

If one hasn't played tennis for years, then plays a vigorous game, the tennis-playing muscles may ache at first. This is not a sign to give up tennis but rather a sign that one should play less long and more often. This calls to mind the boy who combed his hair only once a year, it was so painful he couldn't understand how anyone could stand to do it once each day. Older mothers may be less flexible. Or it may not be age at all but type of activity. The prim secretary who has worked in an office for years with her legs crossed, sitting in a chair, will find that she is stiff and some muscles complain when she first starts her squatting exercises, regardless of her age. This does not mean she can't be a mother; it means her daily activity now, in pregnancy, must include the mother-like squat position at short intervals. These intervals can gradually be lengthened each day as the muscles regain their lost flexibility.

I recall one lady, years ago, who decided frantically at near menopause in her late forties that she had missed something by never having had a baby. This was brought to her with a jolt when her menses became irregular—the first sign to her that her days of fertility were numbered. Her life had been so busy with her career that she hadn't paid much attention to having a baby; that is, until the warning sign appeared that soon she couldn't. That did it, she wanted one, right away!

Her first question, "Do you think I'm too old to have one?" I assured her that, with a bit of assistance, her body could be conditioned adequately to give birth. It would take a bit of doing, for she was overweight, had borderline blood pressure, varicose veins, and poor circulation in her legs from years of office work. Nevertheless, it could be done.

It is true that the ideal *physical* age to give birth is about fourteen years of age. This is not the ideal psychological, spiritual, or economical age, but it is physically. Pregnant girls this age do not really need additional instructions in exercises. Why? They've been doing them anyway without instructions—tailor sitting, squatting, pelvic rocking, regular vigorous physical expenditure of energy in many ways. Even just talking on the phone in the privacy of the home teenagers go through practically the whole gamut of our approved body positions before the conversation is over, as their parents can inform you. I have had obstetrical cases from eleven years of age on up; their problems are many, but none are related to muscular rigidity.

Well, we laid down the law to our middle-aged career woman with no ifs or maybes. She was sincere and so was her husband. It took about every trick in our infertility bag of tricks, but we were blessed with success. Her husband was given an extra dose of coach instruction and the impression that we meant business. She was never to sit in a chair. She was never to cross her legs. She was never to bend her back when she could have bent her legs. She was placed on a low salt, high protein, low carbohydrate, low fat diet, and she stuck to it. Results? During the course of her pregnancy her body fat gradually disappeared, her blood pressure came down to normal, her circulation was better established in her legs, and she performed in labor as efficiently as a teenager. Her posture was improved and she actually sparkled with joy. Her husband sobbed with happiness at the sight and sound of their baby at birth. He kept saying "I thought I would never see one of my own." There wasn't a dry eye in the room from empathy over these people's happiness. She never had another menstrual period afterward—it was to be their only child, but it was a good one. That was ten years ago. Their daughter is a lovely dark-haired girl with large dark eyes and comes by the office regularly to say hello.

The personal rewards of obstetrics are multiple. Obstetricians jokingly maintain to other specialists that ours is the only creative aspect of medicine; the rest is just repair work!

You don't have to be a teenager to do natural childbirth, but the older you are, the more you need its benefits.

3. *Pelvic rocking.* If your wife was instructed in horizontal pelvic rocking (humping and sagging her low back rhythmically while on hands and knees), then came home and performed without your having had any preliminary concepts, you'd think the old girl has lost her mind; she thinks she's a four-legged animal and is down on all fours wagging her tail!

We want you as a husband to know why she is doing this, not only to keep you from institutionalizing her but so that by understanding *why* you will, as a coach, jolly well see to it that she does it. The exercise may look goofy but it actually isn't. It's very logical and very practical. Why?

Let's start from scratch and reconsider a few facts. We are

studying lower animals to see if we can glean from them how it is possible for them to give birth spontaneously without medication. The anatomical differences between people and, say, cats, dogs, horses, and cows are relatively trivial. The anatomical similarities are so remarkable that as premedical students we can study their bodies to gain knowledge about our own.

Having been reared in a farming environment with familiarity of these species, I cannot recall ever seeing varicose veins, swollen ankles, hemorrhoids, fallen wombs, or convulsing mothers among animals. These things I first met in the study of human beings. If their bodies are so similar in structure to ours, why don't they have these things? Why do not the milk cow's hind legs swell and get broken-down veins as she bears calves repeatedly each fertility cycle? I wonder what your wife's body would eventually look like if she also bore a child repeatedly every cycle from the onset to the cessation of her fertility?

What's the main physical difference between these animals and your wife? Somebody taught your wife at a very early age to walk on her hind legs, that's what. Her internal organs are all still suspended in ligamentary little hammocks from her backbone, just like the four-legged animals. These internal organs include her baby box—the uterus—which is suspended from her low back (sacrum) by the uterosacral ligaments. When the backbone is parallel to the ground these organs fall freely forward. When the backbone is perpendicular to the ground, the organs fall downward and inward where, frankly, they weren't designed to be. The heavy, enlarging uterus compresses the blood vessels and interferes with circulation to the legs and kidneys. It stretches its own supporting ligaments out of shape and weakens the back at their point of attachment. A woman has been defined as a biped with a backache, and she has reasons! The nonpregnant uterus weighs about one-half to three quarters of a pound. In the short course of nine months it and its contents increase in size until it weighs fifteen to twenty pounds. This means the ligaments attached to the low back are going to be calling on the spinal muscles of this area to do twenty times more work in these short nine months.

Now, if the leg muscles were to be called upon to run twenty times farther or faster at the end of a nine-month period, how would an athlete prepare them? By binding them with Mr. Goodyear's rubber bands? By trying to do their work for them? Would that tend to strengthen them steadily? Of course this is ridiculous. Doing their work for them would tend only to weaken them progressively as it would any muscle anywhere.

Then what in the world is the logic behind girdles and corsets designed to do the work of the uterine-supporting muscles? Aren't they equally ridiculous and don't they serve to progressively weaken muscles that should be progressively strengthened?

In our office the word *girdle* is a swear word. Recognizing the abysmal insanity of fads and customs, we only scream in protest the first time a woman wears one. From that point on we either swear, weep, or both if we find them again.

Now, if your wife has a physical deformity of her back or abdomen and an orthopedic specialist has perscribed an orthopedic artificial supporting device for good sound medical reasons, that is another matter. What we are dealing with here is healthy women.

Let's use your grandmother as an illustration. If not yours mine will do nicely.

When she was young her back muscles needed no help. Then she began wearing girdles—at first lightweight, not very strong ones. As the years went by, her muscles progressively weakened from the effect of the rubber bands doing their work for them. The next time she bought one it had to be a little stronger, and the next time a little stronger, and so forth, *ad infinitum*, until eventually she ended up with a powerful, big corset that Mr. Goodyear's products couldn't handle alone; it needed whalebone stays and steel rods to assist. Grandmother had to have assistance to lace herself into this awful contraption in order to sit erect in church for one hour. Her back and abdominal muscles were so weakened she couldn't sit erect that long without aritficial support. Comfortable contraption? Try one on some time, gentlemen, and see how you feel! (See Cartoon.)[2]

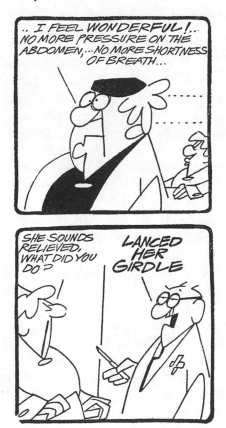

The minute grandmother came home from church the first thing she wanted was to take off her corset; you can't blame her, they're miserable. When she did, her shape suddenly changed. Her abdomen flowed out and over like a skin bag full of water—suddenly released. Where were the abdominal muscles? Long

[2] "Doctor Is In." Drawn for *The Ama News* by Dave Harbaugh.

gone. At church she seemed always attentive, sitting briskly erect as if a board were strapped to her back. Heavens, she couldn't sit any other way. Is this the destiny of your wife?

Let's get back to that athlete who needs to strengthen his leg muscles to do twenty times more work. How will he do it? Not by rubber bands but by exercise, daily, regular exercise. Each day he would exercise a little longer, each time to the point of full fatigue. Each day the muscles would get stronger and stronger. Each day the point of fatigue would get farther and farther along. The blacksmith develops such strong bicep muscles by using them daily, not by squeezing them daily with rubber bands. The same advice goes for your wife's back and belly muscles—she should use them! not squeeze them!

The pelvic rocking exercise, on all fours, serves a double purpose. It makes a temporary four-legged animal out of a two-legged one, and it actively exercises the low back and abdominal muscles which need to be strengthened to support the increasing weight of your offspring growing in her uterus.

If this is your wife's first pregnancy she is to perform this exercise just prior to retiring each night—until the beginning of the seventh month. From that time on she is to do as women who have had previous children do from the very first knowledge they're pregnant: perform it at midmorning (10 A.M.), after lunch (at noon), and midafternoon (3 P.M.) *as well as* before retiring. If she is employed away from home during the day, we know she can't perform during working hours. Employed pregnant wives should do pelvic rocking as soon as they get home, before preparing your meal. After each episode of pelvic rocking they are to lie down in the "running position" on their side, top leg drawn up, back curled comfortably forward, to let the heavy uterus remain forward for a rest period of ten minutes at least, or longer if they are tired or not pressed for time. How long should your wife do this pelvic "tailwag" (it is an up and down variety, not back and forth)? During the busy daytime episodes we usually specify forty wags. At bedtime this number should be doubled with a rest period between the wagging episodes by letting her hips recline against her heels, hands and arms folded before her as a pillow for her head. This is called the "froggy" position of rest. It is actually quite comfortable and is the position babies frequently assume in their crib—bottoms up, head to one side, knees drawn all the way up, hands above or under head. One of our teenage mothers found it so comfortable she dozed off and awakened the next morning still in the same position. Most older women will feel muscle-stretching sensations in their thighs and hips in this position and should stay this way just long enough to catch their breath, then get back up on all fours (hands and knees) and pelvic rock again, forty more rocks, then crawl into bed.

In my early years of practice I used not to specify the number of pelvic rocks, insisting that the patients should do it to the point of tiredness then quit. I altered this suggestion when I got a phone call at midnight from one of our teenage patients. She said, "Doc, I've been doing pelvic rocks since nine o'clock but I'm not tired. Shall I keep it up?" Youth is a wonderful thing, isn't it? Our older patients or long-time secretaries may find fatigue at first before they reach the prescribed number. Of course it's all right to stop and rest when tired. The back muscles will gradually strengthen with time, regardless of age, until the less limber are as capable as the rest.

The purpose of longer bedtime pelvic rocking is to counteract the erect posture during the day, and to bring the uterus forward and upward from where it has descended. The other purpose of deliberately tiring these muscles at bedtime is obviously that she gets to rest afterward. Pelvic rocking need not be done on arising, as sleeping in the running position with the upper leg drawn up serves a similar purpose of allowing the heavy uterus to fall freely upward and forward. This is manifested by the decrease in swelling of the ankles and veins of the legs during the night.

Wayne Wright, the husband of one of our enthusiastic young patients, Carol Wright, an acrobatic dancer, proved his wife had paid close attention at the prenatal class where we stressed complications following the descent of the uterus. He brought in a picture he took of his wife on her due date, dressed in ballet leotards, walking around the kitchen at home—on her hands! Her graceful young body was quite capable of this even at full-term pregnancy.

If I were tired of being a teacher of natural childbirth, I would limit my practice of obstetrics to professional dancers. You should see them perform in labor! Magnificent breath control, relaxation, etc.—old stuff to them. This girl pouted because I wouldn't let her walk back from the delivery room on her hands! She could have, and would have. The only reason I didn't allow it was the inevitable resentment from medical colleagues against our enthusiastic, exhibitionistic natural childbirth patients. They create enough attention just walking back on their feet!

Our suggestion: You get in bed each night before your wife does. It doesn't matter how late it is or how tired she may claim to be; don't let her in bed with you until she does her pelvic rocking!

In summary, this hands-and-knees exercise looks strange but is temporarily making a four-legged animal out of your two-legged one who has been parading around on her hind legs all day, although her internal organs are designed and supported like those of four-legged animals! Evolution hasn't caught up here as yet. In order to prevent the development of varicose veins, chronic back strain, fallen womb, toxemia of pregnancy from decreased kidney circulation, etc., all of which is peculiar to the erect posture, see to it that your wife performs this exercise as directed.

4. *Sleep position.* Again this could hardly be called an exercise, but it is so important we include it for emphasis.

One of our new patients complained of inability to sleep because her husband insisted she sleep on her back so she wouldn't squash the baby. She was miserable with a backache. Let me strongly re-emphasize that a mother cannot hurt a baby in the uterus by lying on it. It's the other way around. The baby *can* hurt the mother by lying on her, especially as it gets larger. Babies are suspended in salt water, which serves as an equalizer of pressure. Any local pressure applied to a bag of water is immediately distributed equally and therefore harmlessly diminished—I believe it is a principle in hydraulics. To illustrate this, one can fill a large, tough balloon full of water, insert an inflated small, fragile balloon inside of it, then try to break the small one by striking the large one. Now, of course, if you strike hard enough you can injure the large one. Or putting it another way, you can hurt a mother, but it is indeed hard to hurt a baby. Even most nonpregnant women sleep on their abdomen or curled up in a ball on their sides. During the early months of pregnancy they should continue the same way. Those who sleep directly on their abdomen will find, as pregnancy progresses, they are trying to balance themselves on a lopsided mountain. The side position with the top leg drawn up and, especially in later pregnancy, supported on something is the preferable position. This "something" to support your wife's raised leg can readily be your own legs or perhaps an extra pillow. Sleeping on your side with your back against your wife's abdomen is not only convenient for her but also allows you to feel the movements of your baby during the night. I find husbands intrigued by this movement if it is a first baby. The intrigue seems to fade with increasing numbers of children, probably related to increased need for rest. Having children is indeed hard work, but nothing compared with taking care of them. I have often joked with my patients that I've "had" about seven thousand but, thank goodness, didn't have to take care of them.

From the waist up we are not so concerned what position your wife assumes in sleep. From the waist down we are very concerned that she draw her top leg up and shift her hips over so she deliberately lies on her baby without hesitation.

Some wives prefer to sprawl with their arms, others prefer to cuddle them under their head or shoulders—it doesn't particularly matter.

The purpose of the drawn-up leg is to form a bony supporting "tent" between the leg bone, hip bone, and bed. This allows the uterus that has been "tail-wagged" out of the pelvis to fall freely away and forward and remain there during the sleeping hours.

In the later months of pregnancy you can realize how uncomfortable your wife would be flat on her back by imagining yourself trying to sleep in that position with a bowling ball lying on your abdomen. I think you would tend to turn on your side so the bowling ball would fall away from you.

Pregnant animals seldom show retained water in their body tissues, whereas pregnant humans do. This can come from too much ingestion of salt or other interference with kidney function. One way of interfering with disposal of water via the kidneys is for a pregnant woman to sleep on her back with her baby on top of her. It doesn't even have to be a baby. Tests were done on urine volume output in women whose uteri were enlarged due to fibroid tumors and not pregnancy. The volume of urinary output was measured in the two different positions and found to be diminished whenever the woman lay on her back. Again, I know of no pregnant animal that spends the night balanced on her backbone with all four legs pointing skyward. This may be a factor in the absence of "toxemia" of pregnancy in lower animals.

Your sprawled-out pregnant wife may leave you only the edge of the bed to occupy as she raises that top leg upward. Don't argue with her; try to adjust yourself to her position, not vice versa.

5. *Legs-apart (abduction) exercise.* In anticipation of this event a daily exercise is suggested for your wife to strengthen the "abductor" or legs-apart muscles. Have her lie on her back, temporarily, with her knees up. You, as a husband, place a hand on the outer surface of each of her knees and exert *mild* pressure

to tend to hold her knees together as she uses her thigh muscles to push them apart. Your hands offer the resistance necessary to strengthen her abductors. Now, your biceps are far stronger than her abductors, so don't build up your masculine ego and use so much force she can't get her thighs apart. Rather use just enough resistance so that with her feet together she can gradually open her thighs to their maximum distance against your resistance. Do this about three times a day.

Here we need the husband as part of the exercise itself. If you look at a bony human skeleton you will notice the wide vacant area between the upper portion of the thigh bones. In the living person this area is filled with the powerful, thick adductor muscles. These are the muscles that pull the legs together. On either male or female they are much stronger than the opposing group that pull the legs apart (abduction), which are located on the outside of the thigh bones. This gaping space between the legs of the skeleton is actually no space at all in the living woman; it is filled with the adductor muscles, which, if her legs are together or even only parallel, completely close off the baby door. To get these muscles out of the way of the baby your wife must be able to "abduct" or pull her legs wide apart. The muscles which perform this are by comparison very weak. The adductors that pull the thighs together are very strong (if anyone has put a scissor hold on you in wrestling you'll notice their power).

The farther apart your wife can pull her thighs in the act of birth, the more room the baby has and the easier its passage is accomplished—for both the baby and the mother. (See Chapter 5.)

6. *"Baby door" muscle (Kegel or pubococcygeal) exercise.* You can check on your wife's progress in learning control of the muscle of the vaginal opening through which the baby actually passes by having her alternately tighten and loosen this muscle after intercourse prior to your withdrawal.

She must learn to do this exercise herself and preferably by listening to another woman describe it to her at exercise class. If no classes are available in your locality, she can learn it by analyzing the muscle action of stopping and starting urination. This is best done on arising when her bladder is full. The pubococcygeus muscle passes, as the name implies, from the pubic bone in front to the coccyx or tailbone in back. It is circular or sphincteric in action and serves to close off or open the three apertures in your wife's bottom: the bladder opening in front, the rectal opening in back, and the baby opening between these two. The same muscle controls all three; they cannot be controlled separately (see Chapter 5). Your wife should deliberately become consciously aware of the difference between tightness and looseness of this muscle so that she can welcome her baby with an open door policy during the act of pushing the baby out. Like any other muscle it will become more flexible and more functional with exercise.

There are other purposes besides proper control at the actual moment of birth. The abdominal muscles are stretched carrying the baby, and this Kegel muscle is stretched having the baby. It is important after the pregnancy and birth that these two sets of muscles be actively exercised to draw them back to their original shape and ability to function.

For years we have fussed at women to do abdominal exercises to draw their waistlines in after the pregnancy is over. It is obvious from a block away if they don't. The Kegel muscle is not so obvious but every bit as important, if not more so, as it is involved in bladder and rectal continence or control in the postpartum.

Many people confuse natural childbirth with unattended (and therefore unmedicated!) childbirth such as grandmother had out on the farm during a blizzard when the doctor couldn't get there to "give her something." She had *unattended* childbirth, not what we are dealing with here. The only similarity is that both lack medication, but there's a whale of a difference between the two! Grandmother was not taught muscle control, for instance. After several unattended births without any program of muscle conditioning before, during, or after, she frequently developed inability to control her urine, especially with a full bladder, upon coughing, sneezing, lifting, etc. This also may have altered rectal control. If you don't believe this, have your wife ask her! The second reason for keeping this muscle in good flexible condition by regular exercise during pregnancy is to better its ability to return to normal function after your wife has babies. (See Chapter 10.)

During pregnancy our nurse teachers encourage our patients at class to exercise this muscle regularly and daily during periods of physical inactivity—e.g., while reading, sewing, watching TV, etc. One clever teacher practices and suggests exercising the Kegel muscle while driving a car—during the periods you are stopped at a red traffic light and waiting for it to change. She also suggests to the group to exercise it at cocktail parties when the conversation is boring. This is one natural childbirth exercise your wife can do in public; nobody will notice!

The third reason for maintaining proper tonus of this muscle is that it seems to be important in maintaining the ability to achieve vaginal orgasms. Postpartum frigidity problems in some instances are related to loss of sensation due to the flaccid condition of this important muscle.

7. *Relaxation practice.* This is our final exercise in which you play a role. There are many other exercises your wife will learn at class, or from books, for her to perform—e.g., how to rise, lift, get to the top shelf in reaching, vertical pelvic rocking, etc. She should adapt each one to her daily activities. If she has impaired circulation in her legs from heredity, previous poor habits, or whatever, there are special exercises in addition to cover this; these she can do without your help.

As I said, relaxation is hardly an exercise—it's more like nonexercise—but must be practiced to be perfected, like all physical acts. As you have read in previous chapters, it is impossible to relax the body without simultaneously relaxing the mind. Here you as a coach can achieve results where none other can. We have been unable to find a coach comparable to a husband, whose familiar pattern of action is essential to mental disassociation and physical relaxation by his wife, during the intermittent pulling sensations of uterine contractions in first-stage labor. In careful anticipation of this you should establish your own pattern of verbal suggestion in short periods of concentrated relaxation, at home daily during the course of pregnancy.

It could be done any time, but perhaps the best time is when the daily chores are done, the other children are in bed, the cat has been put out, the outside doors locked, the lights turned off. In other words, your wife should not be distracted by thinking of chores left undone. She should be able to drift off to sleep lulled by the sound of your voice. First-stage labor is sleep imitation and the time to rehearse it is in bed just before going to sleep. Don't disrupt the program by her having to get up and finish some chore.

Of course she should do her pelvic rocking first. We suggest having a soft throw rug next to the bed so her knees won't be uncomfortable. After pelvic rocking she should curl up on her side, top leg raised (with or without a pillow support—whichever she prefers) and snuggle down into her chosen favorite position for sleep—make her "nest." Your task now is to massage her low back area. These nightly back rubs will endear you to her—they make her feel so good. The uterine muscle is attached in the area of the hollow of her back, the saddle area. Have a can of talcum powder or, if she prefers, her favorite cosmetic skin lotion to lubricate your hands to avoid friction. Use the heel of your hand in a rotary rhythmical motion with fairly firm steady pressure. Let her suggest the details of how and exactly where to rub.

After the back rub combine verbal and touch suggestions of relaxation by whatever combination you two find effective. This varies considerably with every couple, so work out your own. Some wives like to have their husbands hum to them while relaxing; others' hair would stand on end in tension if their husband hummed. Your wife may like familiar repetitive love talk that would be utter nonsense to an outsider but gives her a feeling of security and "he loves me" reassurance. As you start this verbalization give her the reminder "when your uterus contracts this is what we'll do." Simultaneously by direct light touch suggest areas of relaxation, progressively, starting with eyelids, face muscles, lips parted, neck, shoulders, arms, hips, legs, feet. With one hand lightly resting on her abdomen, give it a gentle tap at the moment of inspiration. This is to remind her to "bulge" her abdomen out to draw air in her lungs, then to peacefully let go for expiration—she doesn't have to force air out, it goes out all by itself if she lets go. Her breathing should be peaceful, deep-sighing sleep breaths performed rhythmically.

Some mothers like to have narrative-form talking during the relaxation, describing some previous happy shared trip—"Remember when . . ." This probably relates to deep subconscious security feelings from being read to or being told stories at bedtime in early childhood and is quite useful with some mothers. Work out your own individual pattern and then repeat it each night. Repetition helps. Remind her, "After the nurse is through in the hospital, here's what we're going to do, you and I, when your uterus is working." As she gets drowsy and drops off to sleep, join her—and pleasant dreams of parenthood to you both.

7

Psychological Rules, or How to Live with a Pregnant Wife

WHILE PERFORMING CIRCUMCISION on newborn boys I usually get a reaction out of the female nurse assisting by complaining pseudo-bitterly of a man's lot in life. Women have it easy! All they have to do is menstruate and have babies. In this vale of tears men were born to suffer! Circumcised when we're born, prostate trouble when we're old, and in between we have to live with pregnant women. And that takes a bit of doing.

This line of guff doesn't get me overwhelmed with sympathy from the nurse, but it does evoke some rather emphatic opinions, sometimes vividly expressed.

Let us suffer in silence from the circumcision and prostate problem but explore in detail the problem of living with pregnant women. Let's face a fact: they're nuttier than a fruitcake! But we love them and they're here to stay, so let's learn to live with them.

A pregnant woman is a changed and ever-changing woman. She gradually not only looks different but she feels different and acts different.

Since the mind cannot be separated from the body, the physiological changes in her body affect her mind in certain subtle ways. As her constant companion you should know and understand these ways and adjust your way of thinking and acting accordingly. Your job is more than just planting the seed. You must now tenderly nurture it, cultivate it properly, and not let weeds of anxiety, self-doubts, or unresolved hostilities spring up. Pregnant women, coached by natural childbirth-oriented husbands, sparkle with the joy of life. The little nuisances of physical discomfort from their enlarging abdomens are jovially taken in stride as necessary nuisances without becoming all-encompassing.

What changes can you expect in your wife and what is your role in them?

First and foremost she is not in a "delicate condition" when pregnant. She does not have to discontinue all the activities she found pleasure in before becoming pregnant. She does tire more readily and cannot accomplish as much, but she can still do the same type of things. Growing a baby in the uterus takes energy from her reserve supply. She can't bowl as many games or swim as many laps in the pool as she did before. But she can bowl and she can swim when pregnant, and she should be allowed to participate in practically anything physical that she could do before. The only exception I can think of, offhand, would be high diving in the later months of pregnancy. She can ski, she can skate, she can ride a horse, if she has previously done these things. But if she has never ridden a horse before, this would be a silly time to learn. The same goes for skiing or skating. We have had pregnant rodeo queens who participated in rodeos during their pregnancy. But they had learned to ride a horse before they learned to walk!

Dismiss from your mind the idea that if your pregnant wife fell down during skating, skiing, etc., that she would hurt her baby. Of course if she doesn't know how to fall correctly she can hurt herself—just as she could when she's not pregnant. In my career I have never known a mother to have harmed a baby by any external trauma. The salt water in which the baby is floating equalizes local pressure.

This idea of falling down and thereby losing a baby is a superstition that probably began with the movie *Gone with the Wind*.

Rhett Butler gave his wife a shove at the top of the stairs. She gracefully tumbled down the stairs and conveniently (for the plot) had a miscarriage at the foot of the stairs. Immediately thereafter doctors' offices and hospital emergency rooms were mobbed with out-of-wedlock pregnant women who were battered black and blue and sore but still very much pregnant! It won't work.

If your wife loves swimming, let her swim any time during her pregnancy. Swimming is an ideal sport for pregnant women for many reasons. Suspended in water in any position, except flat on her back, her uterus is deflected upward and out. Also expert swimmers are ideal natural childbirth performers in labor.

The first patient in our series to label the method "painless childbirth" was a swimming instructor. She made me look foolish when I brought in some medical students and doctors who wanted to learn the techniques of coaching a woman in labor. I was going to check her over during first-stage labor and correct her errors. We never expect any woman to be perfect the first time in labor. I hadn't checked this mother yet so I expected, as usual, to give directions and coach. This turned out to be one of the few times when the instructor couldn't open his mouth. There wasn't anything to correct! She had been propped up in the contour chair by her husband, who was perched on the end of the bed. He had drawn the bed tray across the space between her abdomen and thighs and they were calmly engrossed in playing cards.

I announced that with her next contraction I would check her over and correct her errors for the benefit of the medical observers. She smiled cooperatively, and when the next contraction began she said "excuse me a minute" to her husband, laid her hand of cards down on the tray, settled back with her arms on the supporting pillows, closed her eyes, and began the most perfect wave of total relaxation I have ever seen—reflected first in her face, then her neck, and on downward. Her breathing was perfect, deep automatic abdominal or diaphragmatic. The more I checked, the more obvious it was that I couldn't offer a word of advice; she was perfect!

In bewilderment I asked, when the contraction was over and she had picked up her hand to resume playing, how come she was so perfect. She laughed at my puzzled face and mischievously said, "Why, Doctor, I've been teaching this myself for seven years. There's nothing to it!"

I looked even more bewildered and blurted, "You've been teaching natural childbirth?"

She said, "Well, not by that name, but it's the same thing. I'm a swimming instructor and this is the same thing as floating in water!"

I had never before thought of this similarity. My pupils have taught their teacher many times since. What does one do in water to float? Relax completely, breathe gently from your abdomen, leave your eyes closed, lips parted, and breathe through your mouth. She was right. Could the fatal accidents to good swimmers who develop a leg cramp be related to inability to relax totally? You should have seen her hold her breath in second stage as she joyfully pushed into the world a healthy eight-pound baby.

Your wife doesn't have to be a swimmer to have a baby by natural childbirth. As the psychiatrist said, You don't have to be crazy to be a psychiatrist but it sure helps.

No, your pregnant wife is not in a delicate condition. Once a week we beg you to date her and participate in the same sport you two shared when she was not pregnant. If she gets tired, it's a good healthy physical tiredness; it won't hurt her. She will want to rest sooner. Let her. The tiredness most women complain of when you come home from work is not good physical exhaustion that follows doing something physical, accompanied by deep full breathing. Housework does not come into this category; she *has* to do that. But she *gets* to swim or bowl or dance. There is a difference. If you have other children, for heaven's sake get a baby sitter once a week and get her away from them. It's good for *them* too. They get sick and tired of looking at her all the time; they'd like to see someone else once a week. Conversely, if you think a parent doesn't get sick and tired of looking at the same children all week (even if they're perfect angels, which in healthy children isn't likely), stay home with them by yourself one week. I think all husbands would understand a housewife's psychological boredom far better if they "took over" completely one week out of each year. It isn't that it's hard work; it's just repetitious and boring.

Also our problem today is different from Grandmother's day because of higher levels of education. Today wives and husbands are equally well educated; in fact sometimes the wives have gone further in higher education. If their only contact during the day is with their small children, they are bound to feel frustrated. Have you ever tried to carry on an intellectually stimulating conversation with small children?

You go to work at an office. All day you probably meet and deal with people on an intellectual level comparable to your own. When you get home at night you may be tired, but don't be like the usual unthinking husband. Don't just sit in silence and eat the fine dinner your wife has prepared, watch TV until you get sleepy, grunt, and go to bed. How many jittery, nervous women have wailed tearfully, "If he would only talk to me." Have some intellectual pursuits in common with your wife—have something stimulating to tell her about your day's activities. She *needs* to talk and be talked to.

Let's dispose of another widespread misconception—that pregnant women mustn't travel. This ancient superstition dates back to the horse and buggy days; the springs in those buggies were not comparable to present-day cars. I sincerely doubt that even the jouncing of the buggy ever made a mother miscarry. She would have miscarried anyway.

We do advise that traveling a long distance (more than one hour away from the hospital) should not be done in the last six weeks before the due date. It also should not be done at any other time of pregnancy if there is vaginal bleeding and/or cramping. Why? For the simple reason it's deucedly unhandy to have a miscarriage or a baby out on the highway, miles away from medical care. God *only* knows when your wife is going to have a baby. That assigned calendar date is utterly meaningless except as a rough guess. I've never met a baby who could read a calendar. Stay home or nearby in the last six weeks. Most babies do come after their due dates, but as sure as you plan it that way yours will come early. Highway patrolmen are not eager to act as obstetricians.

Prior to the last six weeks, if your wife is not bleeding or cramping (threatening to miscarry), it is perfectly all right to travel if you'll just observe a few rules of common sense. She should sleep eight or more hours out of each twenty-four. Don't overtire your wife by frantically driving night and day to get somewhere in a big hurry. Start earlier, stop and rest regularly—in a motel or hotel and a real bed—without this silly business of trying to sleep in the car. Take along a sack of her favorite fruit to nibble on while riding. A baby is a perfect parasite and doesn't ask when dinner is ready, but depletes its mother's blood sugar by snacking all the time. So should she, on fresh fruit preferably. If her blood sugar gets low, that pregnant stomach may get motion-sickness. If she is prone to such when not pregnant, have your doctor supply you with one of the excellent anti-motion-sickness pills to take along on the trip—just in case.

Airline stewardesses take care of these details if you travel by air. If your purpose in traveling is just to get there, not to see the scenery en route, it is preferable to travel by air. Even autos with the best shock absorbers bob up and down at high speeds and the heavy uterus is gradually tamped down and deeper into your wife's pelvis. She should, therefore, wear loose-fitting garments so she can sprawl on the seat, with one or both legs tucked up and under her. Make frequent stops to allow her to walk around a bit to relieve pressure discomforts. She should ride in the front seat. Let her drive if she knows how and wants to. The purpose is so she'll know when the curves are coming and by expecting them compensate for them. The sudden unexpected sway makes queasy stomachs. If she likes to travel, then observing these simple rules will make it more enjoyable for her.

Another misconception of pregnancy is that women can't take baths, or at least not in late pregnancy. I can't think of anything more miserable than a woman who can't bathe. Of all the times on earth when she needs a bath it is when she's pregnant. Extra mucous, extra perspiration, extra-tired muscles—a leisurely hot bath treats them all and should be a regular evening ritual, just before retiring, all the way through pregnancy. Heat is a wonderful physical agent to promote relaxation and restore muscles tired from carrying a baby around all day.

The old concept that bath water enters the vagina has been disproved. It was thought this might cause infection in the uterus in the late months of pregnancy as the cervix gradually opens a little after "false labor" contractions appear, any time in the last three months.

This folk philosophy was shown to be wrong in two ways. First, women ignored the admonition not to bathe; they bathed anyway and got along fine without evidence of infection. Second, an enterprising doctor, recognizing this, cleverly tested to see if bath water entered a pregnant woman's vagina. He soaked cotton vaginal tampons in a starch solution, dried them, had the mother insert and wear them each time she bathed. To her bath water she added a few drops of iodine on each occasion.

If the water entered the vagina the starch-permeated tampons would turn blue. They didn't, so let your wife bathe all through pregnancy. She'll be a lot easier to live with.

While we're chasing away ghosts of yesterday let's chase away another one that definitely affects you. The same old concept against bathing was applied to sexual intercourse, which went: "Abstain totally in the last months of pregnancy." Comment: hogwash! This was again based on an old assumption that uterine infection would result. On the surface it sounds reasonable, but in actuality there's one thing wrong with the assumption—it just isn't so!

Pregnant Navy wives whose husbands were at sea had no fewer infections than Air Force wives whose husbands were very much with their wives and who, upon careful questioning, had intercourse regularly all the way through pregnancy.

Now, here again, be sensible. We do recommend continuing relations throughout pregnancy—what a lovely time to make love, you don't have to worry about her getting pregnant. However there are a few don'ts.

Don't lie on top of her, especially in the later months. Remember the bowling ball comparison? She's uncomfortable on her back.

Practically any position except this is all right in pregnancy. You're on your own otherwise. Let your wife decide which she finds comfortable. Don't argue with her! Positions means very little to a man, but very much to a woman. A bit of further advice: be gentle. The vaginal flesh is puffy and sensitive during pregnancy from the circulation changes.

Also some women do not particularly enjoy intercourse during pregnancy, due to psychological reasons. Do not get your male ego hurt if she is not as responsive as she used to be. Physical tiredness may be affecting her too. Be patient. She will be a responsive partner again after pregnancy is over. The increased sensitivity of the vaginal and labial flesh sometimes makes some women more responsive during pregnancy. Don't make an issue of it either way. Also the same woman may react differently during different pregnancies.

Your wife may notice uterine cramps or increased labor-like contractions of the uterus after intercourse. Don't let her be alarmed by these; they are perfectly normal. In fact they are probably beneficial and by stimulating the uterus serve to help soften and make flexible the cervix so it will dilate more effectively during labor.

A tribe of aborigines are said to help their wives out in labor, if the contractions become ineffectual and weak, by having intercourse during labor. I haven't yet found a cooperating hospital in which to try to this experimentally. So far all we have achieved is the husband's presence!

If any other old wives' tales have reached your wife's ear and bother her, by all means talk them over with your doctor. Volumes have been written on the silly superstitions accumulated in folklore about pregnancy. The cord does *not* wrap around the baby's head if the wife reaches up. Paint fumes cannot hurt the baby but may make your wife nauseated if they contain turpentine. This can be prevented by good ventilation, if she likes to paint. Most modern paints have water- or rubber-based solvents and do not bother anyone.

Now there are various nuisances of pregnancy which you should be acquainted with if you're going to learn to live with this somewhat neurotic female. For convenience let's divide them into three separate groups of three months each, representing the three "trimesters" of pregnancy.

First Trimester Changes!

PRESSURE

Your wife cannot carry a steadily enlarging abdomen without feeling it. These pressure pains are more prominent in the first three months due to the fact that the uterus is still small enough to sag down deeply into the bony ring of the pelvis. This is like a cork which is too small for the ring of the bottle mouth and falls into the bottle. As the uterus descends it applies pressure, in the front, to the bladder. This limits the capacity of the bladder and at the same time there is increased urine volume from the baby (your wife literally urinates for two). If you have trouble locating your wife when you come home, just stand by the bathroom door. In a few minutes she'll be either coming or going.

There are little guy ropes attached to each upper corner of the uterus called "round ligaments." They pass from the corners of the uterus into a canal on each side of the abdomen. These canals are identical to the ones through which the male spermatic tubes pass. These ligaments pass down to attachments in the major lips of the vagina, on each side. As the uterus descends it causes these structures to knuckle or bend, which produces a muscle spasm in this area. You may be walking down the street with your wife when she suddenly lets out a yelp, bends over, and holds her side. This is usually the right side (the large bowel occupies the left side of the pelvic ring and displaces the pregnant uterus more to the right), although it could be either side.

Don't try to make her keep walking but steer her over to the shop window and have her bend down to act very interested in something in the window. After a few moments the round-ligament spasm will let up and she can comfortably walk erect again. If she has these at home, a bit of pelvic rocking followed by tailor sitting or lying on her side will relieve it. They are not a sign of something wrong but only a result of walking on the hind legs, when these round ligaments were designed for the all-fours position. Of course if severe side pain persists she should contact her doctor.

In back of the descending uterus is the rectum, and the pressure from constipation can be a nuisance in early pregnancy. The proper treatment is twofold: get her off her feet more, in the approved exercise way, to make the uterus come upward and forward, and, second, see to it that she drinks plenty of water and eats roughage (fresh fruit and vegetables) to keep her bowel contents soft.

To each side of the pelvis are the large blood vessels and the nerves that go to the legs. Your wife may get some degree of swelling of her ankles and distention of veins of the legs, particularly if she is employed. See to it that she does her exercises and gets off her feet regularly at home. Pressure on these nerves results in odd numb or hot sensations running down her hips to her legs. They are transitory and usually come from sitting in one position too long. Remind her to move around more.

She will have a general feeling of fullness in her lower abdomen which becomes a dragging sensation if she doesn't get off her feet at regular intervals.

CIRCULATION CHANGES

As your wife's pregnancy progresses she gradually has more blood circulating through her body, estimated at one third more volume. The veins become more noticeable, larger and bluer, especially when they are near the surface, as in the chest, legs, hands, etc. Incident to the increased circulation she will have increased secretion from practically every gland in her body. This includes the mucous glands, not only of the vagina but of the nose and mouth. She will have more saliva, more perspiration, more congestion in her sinuses. Another gland that increases its output is the thyroid gland in the throat. Your wife may get a feeling of fullness in her throat. She also absorbs extra thyroid secretions from her baby's circulation, which results in more thyroid than usual. What are the effects of extra thyroid? She may feel warm when you and others in the room are cool. She may have palpitations of her heart, which is beating stronger anyway to push extra blood around. She may sit up suddenly in the middle of the night with a heavy sensation in her chest and throat from nervous spasm. This coupled with palpitation of her heart may frighten her into thinking she's having a heart attack. Reassure her, remind her to walk around a bit, and if the weather is decent go to an open window for some big, deep, slow breaths. The feeling will pass. She may have numbness and tingling in her hands as if they are "going to sleep." Reassure her that this is to be expected.

She is receiving more hormones from her own glands and in addition from the donations of the placenta. As a combined result her nerves are on edge; she will be jumpy and high-strung. If you're one of the practical joker type husbands and should sneak up behind her and surprise her, in the nonpregnant state she would smile and say "Don't be so silly." If you tried the same trick in the pregnant state, two things would happen: (1) You'd have to get her down off the chandelier, and (2) You would hear new names for yourself that your mother never thought of.

These periods of excitability alternate with periods of depression—for no particular reason except that she's pregnant. You may come upon her unexpectedly and find her crying. Don't get too insistent about finding out exactly what's wrong. It's pretty hard for her to tell you, for the simple reason she doesn't know anything specific that's wrong! She's pregnant and she just feels like crying and to her that's a good enough reason. Darn those logical men!

Laugh *with* her but never *at* her in pregnancy, or she'll bite your head off. Her sense of humor is depleted in pregnancy or sometimes completely warped. She will get her feelings hurt over something you thought was funny or go into peals of hysterical laughter over something you don't consider funny at all. Don't try to understand her sense of humor, just love her and make her feel how glad you are to have her—even if she does act a little nutty occasionally.

The increased circulation combined with a tendency for retention of salt in the body results in a generalized puffiness of her body. This is more manifest in some areas that are rich in blood vessels—for instance, her gums. She may get sensitive gums and pink toothbrush. She should use a less stiff brush during pregnancy. Her nasal mucosa is puffy and fragile and the tiny distended veins may break if she blows her nose too hard. Or she may see specks of blood in her saliva, drained from the back of her nose, especially in association with a cold. She should avoid blowing her nose whenever possible and, if she must, always blow gently with both nostrils open.

SKIN CARE

Her hair may lose its luster and/or tend to come out more when she combs it. We used to advise pregnant women not to spend a lot of money on expensive permanents, but wait until the pregnancy is over, as the hair consistency is more brittle during pregnancy. Her fingernails may peel or break more easily. Her skin will become quite dry, and she should bathe regularly with some bath oil preparation.

The puffiness is visible in her face, bagginess forms under her eyes, giving her a moon-face appearance. It is thought similar puffiness or water retention occurs internally as well as externally. Swelling or puffiness of the brain may account for her episodes of depression, irritability, and illogical excitation. She's not "kookie", there's a physical reason for her actions and feelings. Don't tell her it's all in her head or her imagination—she'll resent such implications and besides there is a physical cause. We see similar phenomena in the nonpregnant state just a few days before the menstrual period begins. It is called premenstrual tension, and you should learn to handle her with kid gloves during that phase. Women are witches (some husbands may want to spell that with a *b*) one week out of each month when not pregnant, and justly so. Have her cut down on salt intake during that week—it helps reduce the causative swelling.

Her eyes are puffy and swollen internally as well as externally. She gets blurring of vision and has trouble focusing while reading. This will leave after pregnancy and does not necessarily mean she needs refraction correction.

Her fingers may swell, and if her ring begins to get snug she'd better remove it. If she tries to do fine sewing she has trouble due to stiffness of her finger joints. All of this is perfectly normal but is aggravated by salt ingestion. If it becomes exaggerated, hide that salt shaker!

There are three very important areas of her skin, important in the sense that they must be made flexible to allow stretching. From above downward they are: (1) her breasts and nipples, which are going to get larger and the nipple skin darker during pregnancy. On the third day after the baby is born they are going to suddenly get quite a bit larger, as they fill with milk. In preparation for the later need to stretch, the skin should be massaged daily with a lanolin-based cold cream of her choice. Perfumed cream isn't necessary; cheaper hand cream works fine. The nipples should be pulled with cold-cream lubricated hands outward with a "milking" action, a dozen "ouchy pulls" a day. By this is meant pulled with enough vigor to produce a slight degree of discomfort. The friction of pulling tends to toughen the skin as well as make it flexible. Unless your wife is a nudist her nipple skin has not seen the light of day since she was eight years old. When children wear shoes all winter, the skin on the soles of their feet becomes tender and sensitive. When they first rub this skin on the pavement in the spring to go barefoot they walk very gingerly. However, after three months of summer and regular friction the skin becomes tough—they can walk on cinders without wincing.

The friction of rubbing is as important to the nipples as the lanolin applied. Nothing that's painful meets with acceptance for very long. Successful breast feeding depends upon non-tender nipples. We check the nipples regularly during prenatal visits for toughness and flexibility and threaten the patient that we will call her husband for assistance in rubbing her nipples daily if we find them still dry, brittle, and tender. Blond and red-haired mothers with fair, thin skin need more attention than brunettes, we have found.

A small amount of sticky yellow-white secretion may be secreted from the nipples in the later months. It is called colostrum, is perfectly normal, and can be rubbed right back into the skin along with the cold cream as nature's little contribution. The husband's manual or oral manipulation of the breasts and nipples in sexual foreplay is perfectly permissible and probably beneficial throughout pregnancy and later during lactation.

The second area of skin that must be made flexible so that it will stretch comfortably is your wife's abdomen. Cold cream should be applied and worked into the skin daily. This prevents the surface layer of skin from cracking or itching. It does not necessarily prevent the formation of "stretch marks," which seem to be inescapable in fair-skinned mothers. These are the reddish streaks that appear on the lower abdomen, hips, and often outer aspects of the breasts during pregnancy. They will turn a silvery white months after the baby is born and should be proudly worn as "service stripes" of motherhood.

The third area of skin that will need to stretch (later) is, of course, the vaginal area. The vaginal lips should be lubricated daily with lanolin or oil after bathing with soap substitutes. This should be continued even after pregnancy to reduce the irritation of underclothes—to prevent rash and keep the skin tough and pliant.

Soap is a strong alkaline agent and is an insult to human skin, as it tends to dry out natural skin oils. Regardless of the advertising claims for how mild a soap is, or how much cold cream the manufacturer adds, soap substitutes with hexachlorophene are far better, especially for sensitive areas. Such soap substitutes should be used in bathing these three special areas during pregnancy.

QUEASINESS

Probably the peskiest nuisance of the first trimester is the queasy feeling. This is related to constantly lowered blood sugar due to the parasitic demands of the baby upon your wife's circulating blood. Later on, her body will compensate for this new demand and release extra glycogen into the blood from liver storage quantities. The body seems slow in calling out the reserves though, and she will be "icky" to some degree during the first three months.

By "icky" we mean lightheaded, shaky, dizzy with nausea or a squeamish feeling in her stomach. If she ignores these signs and doesn't replenish her blood sugar, they can go on to a black-out feeling or even actual fainting or severe nausea with vomiting or both. The treatment is based on the baby's wanting and taking nourishment from her blood stream every hour on the hour, day and night. The baby is selfish and demanding in his dependency. He takes whatever he needs whenever he needs it. He doesn't ask Mama first if she can spare it. He also doesn't starve four hours and then stuff himself for a few minutes as adults are accustomed to do. As a result there are three commandments of pregnancy regarding *how* to eat, which you should see that your wife observes. The troublesome "queasy" feeling will either disappear or be reduced to a minimum.

Wife commandment one. "Thou shalt not let thy stomach go empty."

The pregnant woman should nibble (baby is little and it doesn't take much) between meals on sweets every hour on the hour. This need not mean she will get fat; we said nibble, not stuff. The only approved form of sweets is fresh fruit, in any variety. Frḙsh fruit has a readily absorbed and assimilated form of natural sugar which is converted to blood sugar rapidly, plus beneficial vitamins. She should be a good fresh-fruit shopper and have several varieties available at all times to avoid montony. If she gets stuck away from home and begins to get lightheaded and squeamish, and no fresh fruit is available, as a temporary expedient she'd better nibble on any form of sweets she can find. If she is employed while pregnant she should take along some fruit to nibble on intermittently between meals. Tell the employer it's doctor's orders.

I recall a schoolteacher who continued teaching while pregnant —as well she should. She took a sack of grapes along to school and furtively ate two grapes every hour. She got along fine. One morning, in a hurry, she forgot her grapes and didn't have time to go back for them. She tried to stick it out until noon but didn't make it. She got lightheaded around 10 A.M., vomited at 11 A.M., and fainted at 11:30 A.M.

Most women routinely carry a lower blood pressure than men. Why I don't know. I have various theories about it, but my wife doesn't seem to agree with any of them. Low average blood pressure means longevity (women have a habit of outliving men). Those with low blood pressure should not *suddenly* change from a horizontal to a vertical position (it makes them dizzy), and they should nibble between meals even when not pregnant. Low blood sugar combined with low blood pressure produces a tired, irritable person. In World War II when women first invaded the factories while their menfolk were invading the battlefields it was found that there were fewer accidents and more productive woman-hours if they gave coffee breaks between meals. The benefit wasn't so much the coffee as it was the pastries that accompanied it. Low blood-pressured women were meant to eat lightly and frequently, pregnant or not.

Dismiss from your mind that her nibbling on sweets between meals, especially fresh fruit, will result in your being married to an obese woman. Overweight is more likely to result if she doesn't. Going for long hours empty makes her so frantically hungry that she tends to overeat when mealtime finally comes. An enterprising promoter made a fortune on weight pills to be taken at 10 A.M. and 3 P.M. The pills were remolded hard candy from a leftover Christmas stock, to which he added an insignificant dab of vitamins. He had many testimonials as to their effectiveness. Remember your mother admonishing you not to eat sweets just before your dinner, you wouldn't eat all your dinner if you did! Same principle.

Wife commandment two. "Thou shalt not overload thy pregnant stomach."

There are several reasons for this. One, there isn't as much room. The rising uterus limits the space. Two, there is a delayed emptying time of the stomach in pregnancy from the muscle-relaxing effect of hormones. Food tends to stay there and form gas, especially foods that are slow to digest, such as cauliflower, onions, green peppers, beans, etc. This results in the "heartburn" of pregnancy. Nothing to do with the heart, but it produces gas pressure under the ribs. Any antacid preparation except baking soda may be used to counteract it at the time of discomfort.

Thirdly, sudden high elevations of blood sugar from a lot of food at once will result in a compensatory let-down drop of blood sugar later.

If you take your wife out for a dinner engagement, that's fine. You should do this regularly, as she gets tired of her own cooking, good as it may be. However, during pregnancy take plenty of time, dine leisurely, discuss the European situation or what have you between courses.

Wife commandment three. "Thou shalt not go to bed on an empty stomach—have a protein nightcap."

Grandmother's morning sickness of pregnancy has disappeared since we began insisting on a bedtime snack of protein. Morning sickness was an inescapable result of too long emptiness. Grandmother ate supper at 5 P.M., then didn't eat again until about 6 A.M.—thirteen hours between meals is too long.

The reason for protein food is that it takes longer to convert to blood sugar and the effect lasts longer during the sleeping hours. Let your wife decide which protein. Leftover lean meat, cheese sandwich on whole wheat bread, high protein processed breakfast cereal, etc. Again it doesn't take much, but it takes some.

If your wife gets up to go to the bathroom during the night, and she will, let her nibble on a little something out of the refrigerator before returning to bed. This helps tide her over until morning.

WHAT SHE SHOULD EAT DURING PREGNANCY

Your wife may get bizarre cravings for some ungodly food at some ungodly hour. Quit grumbling, get dressed and go get it! Some pregnancies don't manifest these odd cravings, but then again some do. No one knows why; it's just part of the general picture. Make a joke out of it—laugh, boy, laugh—don't act misused. After all, you may be reminded who started all this business in the first place.

The actual diet your wife should follow will vary with her size and other hereditary factors as an individual and should be supervised by your doctor. In general, as to type of food there are four "no" categories, which we depend upon our husbands to police.

First "no"—salt. Unless you live in a very hot climate and your wife perspires excessively, she does not need to add additional salt to her food. There's enough salt in food the way it comes. In some foods there's far too much—pickles, ham, bacon, potato chips, salted peanuts, and such.

Second "no"—animal fats and oils. Keep them to a holy minimum. Broil that meat instead of frying it. Have her eat the lean part instead of the fat. Get her a special butter dish containing salt-free corn oil oleo instead of butter, and see that she uses it. Fresh vegetables, tossed salads—all she wants, but have her use vinegar, lemon juice, or non-oily low-calorie salad dressing, or mixtures of these, instead of the ordinary mayonnaise and salad dressings. She may prove to be a little sneaky, so keep a sharp eye. Don't be mean, be lovingly firm. Your motivation is how pretty she is and how you want her to remain so. Remind her, gently, of that female acquaintance who used to be so pretty, before she had babies.

Whole milk is unnecessary. Butterfat in any form is unnecessary. Some doctors feel any milk is unnecessary. In contrast to other animal mothers, humans are the only animals who eat baby food (milk) after becoming adults.

No one knows what future investigation may reveal. Maybe nature designed milk as baby food only and never intended it for continuation through adult life, as is true in other than human animals. Until more is learned, let it suffice to drink skim milk, and only a reasonable quantity of that. Some mothers connect milk with motherhood and guzzle a gallon a day. Three glasses is plenty. Calcium is contained in other foods as well as milk. Milk is a cheap source of protein but is grossly overrated otherwise, other than for calves. Don't let your wife worry for fear of not having milk in her breasts if she doesn't tank up on it in her stomach. There is no connecting pipe between her stomach and her breasts. All other animal mothers adequately feed their young at their breasts and *no* other animal mother drinks milk! I have seen women who abhor milk hold their noses and choke it down because they were pregnant. This is ridiculous. If your wife craves milk and likes it, make it skim milk in reasonable quantities.

Third "no"—white flour and its various forms. The brown outer kernel of the wheat seed is taken off and given to cattle in the form of bran and "shorts." The white inner portion consisting mostly of starch and a small amount of protein is ground up to make flour for people because it's prettier. We tend to have healthy cattle and wan people as a result. There are many good *whole* wheat, low caloric products over in the "stay slim" division of the supermarket.

Go shopping with her, take her arm, and steer her firmly down that aisle. When others are eating pastry products between meals she should be nibbling on fresh fruit instead.

Fourth "no"—sugar in its various concoctions. Candy, canned fruit, pastry goods, etc., seem to produce an obsession for more, and more, and more. It's deucedly hard to eat just one piece of candy, or just *one* little sweet roll, or just *one* piece of bread and jelly.

Bees come to our rescue here with their sweet concoction, honey. Chemists have yet to analyze all its contents but, in general, it is used to raise the blood sugar of athletes (swimmers, boxers, etc.) to give them additional energy rapidly. Pregnant women also need additional energy. It is not a matter of calories but of efficient and immediate utilization to produce energy that prompts us to suggest honey as a substitute, whenever possible, for the sugar bowl. Also, for reasons I don't understand, it does not produce that obsession for more, and more, and more. In fact it is self-limiting and will produce nausea if overused.

There are jellies, preserves, soda pop, and so on that are artificially sweetened. Have your wife browse and select down that aisle as well in the supermarket.

In conclusion, let your doctor individualize your wife's diet—everyone's needs are variable. Keep in mind the concept that she is feeding herself, not her baby; he will take care of his own needs automatically. Eliminate from her mind the misconception that how much she eats will affect the size of her baby—this isn't so. It will only affect the size of the *mother*.

Second Trimester

As your wife enters the fourth month of pregnancy you will note a pleasant change of personality—for the better. She looks better. She becomes radiant. She sparkles and is fun to be around. This second three-month period is the most comfortable part of pregnancy.

Why? Many reasons. The queasy feeling is rare because her body is adjusting to that dear little "parasite." The uterus has grown large enough that it doesn't fit in the pelvic ring any more and now is deflected forward instead of downward. This produces the little "O" which is external evidence of fertility now, and a convenient place to rest her book while reading. The pressure pains described in the first trimester have let up. She still gets an occasional round-ligament cramp in her sides, but the pressure is less on all those organs deep in the pelvis. Her personality reflects happiness. We doctors notice it on office calls. Instead of that long list of "what the heck's going on inside me" type of complaint she meets us with a cheery greeting.

It has been said that the only function of the navel is to serve as a repository for salt while eating celery in bed. Nature suggests the abstinence of added salt in the diet by now flattening out the navel so it won't hold salt. The navel will now gradually begin to protrude instead of being inverted.

Her breasts are enlarging and were never more lovely. She will be proud of her figure and she will need an adjustable maternity or nursing bra now.

Anywhere from the fourth to fifth month she will feel the

movement of her baby for the first time. Up to then she has suspected that the rumor she was pregnant was probably true, but this is different! She *knows* she is pregnant now, she can feel the baby kick! It's a delightful feeling to a mother; the wonderment of the miracle of life will occupy her even more.

There is an old rule of thumb that if you add five months to the date she first felt your baby kick it will be the true or more accurate due date. This, the first baby movement, is hard to assess, as the early movements are momentary and she will not be really sure. Then later on, after it is kicking regularly, she will conclude, why, that must have been it last week. Just for fun, arrive at a date when she felt the first real thump (not the flutter which precedes it), add five months and see what you come out with. This supposedly takes into consideration the rate of growth of the individual baby. If it's a speedball in growth and kicks early, it should come early. If it's a slowpoke in growth and kicks its mother late, it should come late. Maybe! There are too many variables involved to be dependable—such as how much salt water is enclosing this particular child, its position in the uterus, etc. But it keeps up your interest. You can make up a "pot" with your wife, relatives, and friends—as you do with World Series scores—and see who wins. I've seen nearly as much excitement from a husband in the delivery room over winning the pot as over having the baby.

You or your wife may notice at times a slow, rhythmical, little jumping motion of her abdomen. It is too slow to be a heartbeat, too regular to be arms or legs moving. What is the baby doing? We've heard that question many times. The baby is hiccoughing. They swallow the salt water they are immersed in and occasionally, just as on the outside, they get hiccoughs.

Your wife is no invalid or in any delicate condition. Parade her proudly, take her out, let her run freely. Now is the time to do the shopping for the baby supplies and plans for his reception. Help her plan and choose the colors or paint the crib and get things ready. After all, it's your baby too, so take an interest.

Make love to her in the car on the way home from the movie—if it's a lovely night. Lover's lane wasn't meant for unmarried lovers only. Variety is the spice of life—locations I mean. Monotony dulls a marriage. Take your wife out, she'll enjoy it.

Charge her storage battery of love. Mother love to a baby has been defined as the gradual release of husband love and affection that was built up and stored from attentions received during pregnancy. Don't get nauseating about it but give her little extras. Tell her how much you love her and show her how much—she never gets tired of being reminded.

Let's add a husband commandment here: *Date your wife at least once a week.* Do the things with her you found joy in sharing before you were married. Why did you pick her as your choice of companion for life? Don't quit living just because somebody put your names on a piece of paper headed marriage certificate. If you have other children, get a baby sitter on this once-a-week occasion. Don't say you can't afford this. There are no reasonable excuses. You can trade around and take turns baby sitting with another young couple of your acquaintance in a similar situation. Money helps, I'll grant you, but what inexpensive things did you do that were fun before you married? Do them again.

And don't tell me you can't spare the time. Take the time! I don't care what sort of work you're in or how hard you're struggling to achieve some goal. First things first, and keeping those home fires burning brightly takes precedence over anything else. Many a man gets so wrapped up in his work that he forgets and neglects the other facets of his role. What does it profit you to "arrive" only to find you have lost your companion somewhere along the road? It can get mighty lonely up there.

Third Trimester

This is the old home stretch. As your wife enters the seventh month her abdomen becomes ponderously heavy. She will have to move around more slowly now. Making the bed, which took five minutes before, now takes fifteen. Get her help with the housework. Do the grocery shopping for her. Carry the heavy loads for her. Send the ironing out or make her do a little every day rather than saving it up—if you can't afford to have it done. As an obstetrician I abhor a pregnant woman ironing for hours. It can hardly be done conveniently in any position except standing. Have you ever noticed a woman's hips and pelvis move rhythmically as she irons? This back and forth movement tamps the baby down deeper and deeper in her pelvis—the exact opposite of the beneficial pelvic rocking.

She will tire more easily now. She will still want to go places, but she won't want to do as much and she'll want to come home earlier.

Why? The uterus is larger and heavier and harder to carry around.

The presenting part of the baby, that part which is coming out first (usually the head), is being pushed down into the pelvic ring by the forces of the uterine muscles contracting. They contract at irregular intervals for irregular durations and this is called false labor or, medically, Braxton Hicks contractions. Such muscular action could be compared to that of a player who after sitting idly on the bench starts warming up in expectation of playing in the game soon. He would run up and down the side lines flexing his football playing muscles, getting them ready.

Your wife's uterus is now doing the same thing—warming up. The football player does not act with as much vigor on the sideline as he will after entering the game. Similarly, your wife's uterus does not contract as hard, or as long, or as often as it will later "in the game." It contracts hard enough, though, to put pressure on her low back and tailbone. It brings back the bladder pressure, rectal pressure, legs swelling, vein swelling, and so forth, described in detail in the first trimester. She must get off her feet more. She must rest more. She must do horizontal pelvic rocking now four times a day, at midmorning (10 A.M.), after lunch at midday, again at midafternoon (3 P.M.) and, of course, at night before retiring. After each pelvic rocking session, she should lie down for at least ten minutes (longer if she wishes) on her side with her top leg drawn up. She should sit or lie down ten minutes or more of each hour if she's at home. If employed, she should seek out a ladies' lounge after lunch, pelvic rock, and rest a few minutes before returning to work.

She can remain active and accomplish a lot of things yet. She should not stay too long in any position, even approved ones, or she'll get stiff and uncomfortable. She will want to be taken out on dates still but not to such formal or long-drawn-out affairs. A good place to take her now is the drive-in movie theater. She can occupy the back seat, sprawled comfortably in a large loose wrapper (and nothing else), tailor sitting, and watch the movie. This is much more comfortable than sitting in public with knees primly together. If you have other children, let them play out of the car in the children's area, but *you*, sir, keep an eye on them.

One of the pleasant aspects after the seventh month is to have you, the husband, listen to the baby's heart beat. The doctor does this in the office and if you wish and ask, he may let you listen through his fetoscope. However, don't be too impressed with his fancy gadget because at home you can hear the baby better than he can by just putting your ear on your wife's abdomen and pressing your ear steadily against the skin. The sounds are diluted in his gadget, but you can hear them directly. The only reason the doctor doesn't listen directly is that it's rather undignified.

Get out your watch, after you have placed your ear at the proper point to hear the sound, and count the number of beats per minute. I would suggest you start your listening on the left side of her abdomen and just a little lower than her navel. Most babies lie with their backs to the left of midline, but not necessarily. If you don't hear it there, let your ear wander around until you do.

What will it sound like? Like a watch ticking. The rate averages 140 per minute but may vary as much as from 100 to 160.

There may be other sounds that confuse you, gurgles and swishes, of intestinal movements or a uterine "soufflé" sound made by the flowing of blood through the uterus. After a little practice you'll be able to distinguish which is the baby's heart sound.

Superstition has it that if the fetal heart rate is over 140, the baby will be a girl. If it is less than 140, a boy. Boys are slow and girls fast, supposedly. Theoretically, if the child will grow to large stature its heart needs to beat more slowly; if destined for small stature, its heart will beat faster. An elephant's heartbeat is slower than a hummingbird's.

Count the heartbeat all you want to, but don't count on the boy-girl prediction. It's all guesswork and fun—like what's in a Christmas present. But you still have to wait for Christmas day to open the gift to see what's in it. Don't get your heart set on one or the other; you may be surprised in spite of heartbeats.

There *is* a way of telling whether it's a boy or girl or not before its birth. A doctor can insert a long needle through the abdomen and uterus and withdraw a sample of the amniotic fluid. It can be spun down in a centrifuge and the chromatic pattern in the cellular debri studied. But who in the world wants to go through all that just to ruin the pleasant surprise of opening your presents at Christmas? Besides, we rather hope you'll accept the baby regardless of its sex. They're a little hard to put back in case you don't want them!

In the last trimester the baby is so close to your wife's rib cage that its movements may give her "pregnancy pleurisy." This is not actually pleurisy but is a sharp twinge under or along her ribs similar to pleurisy. It comes, again, from the pressure of the baby's movements. No treatment is effective except getting her off her feet more often.

Also the pressure upward of the growing uterus will produce a shortness of breath in general and a sudden suffocating sensation occasionally, in particular. This sensation occurs when the baby straightens out his legs and suddenly interferes as the diaphragm is about to descend in inspiration. This gives the same sensation to your wife as if, just as she happened to breathe in, someone clapped their hand over her mouth. She won't really suffocate. If the breathing muscle can't descend at that moment, all she has to do is open her rib cage and chest-breathe or sigh until the baby withdraws his feet.

These baby feet may also temporarily block emptying time of her stomach, and burping and "heartburn" are characteristic results.

Somewhere along the course of the third trimester the baby will "drop" or engage itself in the pelvis. This is not as abrupt as it sounds. Rather the baby sort of settles down at a lower level and keeps gradually getting lower, due to the effect of the downward thrust from gravity and the effect of its own muscle contractions. *When* the baby drops does not denote that labor is due shortly or even correlate with the onset of labor. There simply is no reliable sign that one can depend on to tell when labor will start. If babies were all born an identical size, we could then estimate on that basis. But babies insist on coming in assorted sizes. Perhaps it's just as well because we doctors can't estimate their size accurately anyway. Large, medium, and small is as close as we can come. The passenger won't hold still and manages to elude measurement.

Your wife will occasionally have "hot flashes" in this phase of pregnancy. This is not a sign of the change of life but the effect of the now-large uterus contracting and thereby forcing the blood from its muscles back into the mother's circulation. She feels intermittently warm and then, as the uterus relaxes and the blood runs back, a clammy chilly sensation, momentarily. This alternation of circulation generally also produces brain effects. She may experience panicky feelings—usually manifested by sudden fears that she "can't possibly go through with it." "It" in this case, is all of motherhood—pregnancy, labor, birth, and rearing children. She gets little panicky, trapped feelings, and has doubts of her ability as a mother. Give her a gentle reminder that this feeling has been manifested similarly in all women but they find out later, sometimes to their surprise, that they perform beautifully when the time comes and become admirable mothers.

The same brain phenomena occurring during sleep produces bizarre nightmares during the last three months. Your wife may awaken startled, having dreamed that she had a two-headed calf instead of a baby, or multiple babies—"They couldn't shut them off." The latter phenomenon probably is related to the conscious wondering during the day, "How can one baby have so many feet? It must be more than one." The truth is all the movement that puzzles her is not feet alone; there are hands, elbows, knees, etc., as well as feet. With all this baby activity now is the time to prepare her more carefully for sleep as described in the chapter on progressive relaxation techniques.

We have carefully gone over the details of the nuisances of pregnancy, the little discomforts, pressure pains, etc. This was purposeful in order to acquaint you with how your wife feels during preganancy and why. I firmly believe in the power of positive thinking, so let's wrap it up on a pleasant note.

In spite of all these little nuisances this fertile procreative time is the most pleasant part of your wife's life. The rest of her life she will look back upon these days with tenderness and a fond smile. She will always wish she could live them over again, in spite of the nuisances. I could also give you a list of several hundred sterile women, or women married to sterile men, who would cheerfully give their right eye to trade places with her. They will never know the thrill and satisfaction of being part of the miracle of giving life to a new individual—one that blends the physical and mental inheritances of your respective bodies and souls, manifesting forever your shared love, a new person to carry on where you must leave off, to make the world a better place. The nuisances of parenthood are so few and trivial, the blessings so many and ennobling.

8

"Does My Wife Have To Be 'Cut'?"

A GRANDMOTHER of one of our young mothers was brought forcibly to the office for treatment, sputtering protests. She had an intense distrust of doctors, had never been to one in her eighty years, and was proud of it! She was a rather slight Irish lady with sparkling eyes and peppery spirit. She had a delightful personality, and I took an immediate liking to her. I gently asked what her trouble was and she snapped at me, "Well, sonny, my menstrater has been fallen out for twenty years, what do you think you can do about it?" She used a tone of voice that implied she didn't think I could do a thing about it!

The old lady had a complete prolapse of the uterus, or "falling of the womb" as the condition has been called. I thought Grandmother's new term "menstrater" was a more meaningful word than either uterus or womb. I'm all for including it in the medical dictionary!

I was old enough to be flattered by her derogatory "sonny." My next question brought out the great principle of obstetrical management that this chapter is concerned with. I asked her how many babies she had had. "I had six big babies—all over nine pounds—and I never had any fool doctor cuttin' on me. I had midwives, they knew how to deliver babies without all that cuttin'!"

Grandma was right. Midwives were not allowed to "cut"; that

136

was a doctor's privilege. I have the greatest respect for midwives, then and now. They served a noble purpose in the development of this country and other countries and there are many excellent ones still performing capably in remote areas.

However, I know there are occasions where a little cutting does a great deal of good. No, your wife doesn't *have* to be cut, I think she would *prefer* to be cut. With term-sized babies the cut is beneficial in most instances.

To illustrate my point, I tell patients if they don't want to be cut we will, at their insistence, use the midwife technique of getting a baby out that relatively small opening without cuts or tears.

What was the midwife technique? I'm amazed to find today's childbearing generation hasn't the foggiest idea. Let's study a little history together. Perhaps you have seen movies of olden days—*Gone with the Wind*, for example. The midwife's first request, to all concerned, is for what? Hot water! Not a tea cup full but buckets, tubs, pans, etc. What does she do with all that hot water? I have asked our prenatal classes that question and got quite a variation in answers. "It makes the husband cut wood to keep him out of the way." "It's to make tea for the doctor." No, the midwife puts salt in these steaming buckets of water, then she starts rounding up clean cloths, freshly ironed to sterilize them. She has been known to improvise with her own petticoats in time of need. The cloths are torn into strips and placed in the hot salt water to be used as steaming compresses to be applied to the laboring woman's vaginal area. After one cloth cools down a hot replacement is applied, and so on through the entire course of labor. These hot salt water compresses are alternated with application of olive oil and manual massaging of the vaginal opening to effect stretching. If you have ever soaked some minor infection of your skin in hot salt water for a time you will recall how the skin becomes loose and wrinkled, losing its normal elasticity. This prolonged soaking combined with vigorous manual massage and stretching results in a gaping aperture. The problem is that human flesh, unlike rubber, does not spring back into its original shape. Even the best grade of rubber never quite assumes its original proportions after stretching, and if repeatedly stretched it becomes very flaccid eventually. The same applies to vaginas. All human flesh has a different degree of elasticity, but vaginas, so treated, have a tendency to remain stretched, with the result so well demonstrated by the condition of this dear little misguided lady.

This grandmother was patiently educated about her condition and had a vaginal hysterectomy and plastic surgery to reform her vagina. She was very proud of her new vagina and on her postoperative check mischievously stated, "Sonny, I wish I'd met you twenty years sooner. I'd a landed me another husband."

No, we don't keep buckets of hot water in delivery rooms today, as we've found doing the little cuts called episiotomies prevents overstretching of the vagina. It is true, however, that natural childbirth physical training greatly reduces the need for large cuts and in some more flexible flesh, any cuts. Ours are done just before the baby is born, are the midline variety, and are far smaller than those needed for untrained patients.

Why do humans need these when animals don't? I honestly don't know. I have a pet theory which like most armchair philosophy is probably wrong. I'll give it to you for what it's worth.

The human animal differs from all others in two important respects. It walks erect and wears clothes—or at least some coverup. Even the briefest bikini bathing suit includes a cloth covering of the vagina—on some this is nearly all it covers! We now have "topless" bathing suits but not as yet "bottomless." In the erect postured human animal the sun would seldom shine on the vaginal area even if it weren't clothed. (I have had the privilege of acting as obstetrician for professional nudists, and from the physical standpoint I could not argue with those sun-tanned-all-over mothers. Their skin is more flexible, less brittle.)

The skin around the vagina in nonnudist mothers is usually

brittle and chapped. We apply to this condition the term "panty rash," chapped lips of the vagina regularly irritated by moist cloth and the friction from movement. This is the same condition as "diaper rash" in babies, and "jock-strap itch" in men who perform regularly as athletes. In babies the source of moisture on the cloth is obvious, in men athletes it comes from perspiration, in women, particularly pregnant women, it comes from perspiration and vaginal mucous. Both are normal and profuse in pregnancy. They cause moisture in clothes too close to the skin, which results in chafing and irritation. If a wet cloth were rubbed constantly on the oral lips they too would become chapped and would crack when the dentist says, "Open wide." Animals have an advantage here. Not only is their vaginal area uncovered, they are constantly exposed to the toughening and evaporating effect of sunlight, so they have vaginal skin which is flexible instead of brittle.

If the animals have their vaginas fully stretched having their babies, why don't they get fallen "menstraters" you ask? No four-legged animal gets fallen "menstraters" for the simple reason that gravity makes their organs go up and back into them, rather than down and out, as happens in humans because of the erect posture.

Enough theory, what's the practical application with your pregnant wife? If you want to clear up diaper rash on a baby, remove the diaper, the irritant. Put it on the crib mattress rather than on the baby.

This is also true for women. If you remove the panties, the irritant, you improve the skin. Custom does not work in our favor though, men, and I wish you better luck than I've had. These flimsy garments could not possibly add much warmth, but women seem to have become accustomed to them. We do wish you would encourage your wife not to wear them at all or not to wear them around the house in her ordinary duties. Have her hang them on the hall tree with her hat; put them on, if she must, as she leaves, take them off along with her hat as she returns. Or as a last resort wear droopy old garments that do not fit tightly against the vaginal skin.

The internal vaginal skin is called mucosa and is constantly moist with mucous. This skin does not need cutting as it unfolds quite readily when the baby descends. It is the outer skin which is brittle and needs to be cut. The vaginal mucous is normal and in constant production, although more plentifully during pregnancy as previously mentioned. There is normally no need for douching, as washing out the mucous defeats the purpose for which it exists. Do not inject solutions up your nostrils to wash out mucous either. You wouldn't have a clean nose if you did, but, eventually, an infected, dry, irritated one. The vaginal mucous is in itself clean and cleansing in its action, from above downward. It is there for a reason and should be left alone in healthy women. I enjoy teasing my dentist friend and a friend who is a throat specialist. As an obstetrician I deal with the cleanest opening of the body whereas they deal with the one laden with bacteria. If there is any doubt about this, the study of the stained mucous smear from the respective areas will be very revealing. Normal vaginal mucous contains a single species of bacillus (Döderlein) which maintains an acid reaction that prevents the growth of other bacteria.

In the care of the external skin of the vagina implore your wife to abstain from soap, which tends to remove natural protective skin oils, and to bathe *gently* with soap substitutes containing hexachlorophene. After rinsing and drying gently she should then anoint this area with any lanolin-based cold cream of her choice.

If you are competent as a teacher your wife's flexible skin will need very little in the way of incisions.

When necessary these little cuts (episiotomies) are done in the back corner of the vagina, in the tough flesh that is in front of the rectum. This flesh is tendonous in nature and represents the insertion in the midline of the tendons of muscles that surround the vagina. With the oral lips, chapping is most likely to happen at the two corners of the mouth. The corners of the vaginal lips are front and back. By doing the little incision at the flexible back corner we release tension to prevent any cracks of the skin at the rigid front corner where the vaginal lips surround or house the clitoris. This little bump is the vestigial penis retained from the undifferentiated embryo of all women, and is an important trigger of passion. We do not want scars of cracks or incisions at this corner, as they may interfere with proper response to intercourse later.

Even though we use no anesthetic we make a bet with our mothers that they can't tell their husbands if or when we do this little incision. If they can, we'll refund their fee.

We wink at the husband and show him the scissors at the time we perform it, then after the baby is born ask the mother to tell her husband just exactly with which push we did the cut. We have had to refund no fees because the properly applied pressure, the natural anesthetic, is most effective. After the baby and placenta have been passed, we leisurely inject novocaine in the edges of the cut and put in the few small stitches. The novocaine is necessary then, as the pressure anesthetic is gone.

I recall teasing a doctor's wife to illustrate the effectiveness of God's anesthetic to a group of student nurses and new interns. She was an R.N. as well as a close friend and therefore eligible for teasing. No fee being involved for her as a doctor's wife, in the course of pushing during second stage I made her a bet of fifty dollars that she couldn't accurately tell the ring of observers at what moment I performed the episiotomy. She got a mischievous gleam in her eye and bet she could. I knew what she was basing her confidence on. She had had other natural childbirth babies and she knew that you can perceive additional pressure contact at this area, not pain but pressure sensation. Being a nurse, she also knew where the scissors were kept—in a pan of sterile water nearby.

To fool her I hid an extra pair of scissors in one hand, then with each push simply touched the area, just to confuse her. On one of the pushes I used the hidden scissors and instead of just touching, actually did the incision. It was obvious to the observers she could not tell any difference. On the next push I reached over into the pan, got the regular scissors but just touched her with my gloved hand. She triumphantly informed the audience I had cut her that time, much to their delight. She lost the bet but helped to demonstrate a great fundamental natural childbirth fact: Properly applied pressure prevents pain.

Another illustration came in the form of a letter from a furious former patient. She had had several babies by natural childbirth, then moved to a distant city. She went to a new doctor who practices natural childbirth—only he was one of those who confuses hypnotic suggestion with the physical factors of pain relief. In fact he didn't believe there are physical factors. He obtained the history of her previous episiotomies without medication and learned that she hadn't felt them. This he interpreted as pure mental suggestion. At the birth of the baby he performed the episiotomy at the proper time while she was pushing, but then went ahead and put in the stitches later without novocaine, insisting to her during his action that "it is numb, it doesn't hurt." Her letter was rather vivid: "It hurt like hell!" Properly prepared hypnotic trances can produce analgesia by suggestion. With this I have no argument, but do not confuse this with the physical facts of natural childbirth. I have used both approaches and found that the simplicity of natural childbirth compared to the complexity of hypnosis is like wheeling up a cannon to shoot a sparrow when a BB gun would have sufficed.

In summary, do not let your wife build up a mighty issue over these simple little cuts. If she fell down and cut her knee in a similar way, she would go to the doctor and he would inject novocaine around the edges of the cut and hold it together with a few simple stitches. She would pay little attention to the whole thing. The cut made for having a baby is in a different location but similar in nature and management. The main difference between the two actually is that the cut at the "baby door" will heal remarkably faster and with far less discomfort. The extra circulation associated with pregnancy promotes more rapid healing. The Creator is very efficient.

9

When Will the Baby Come?

The question can be accurately answered in three words: "God only knows." As doctors we are far more concerned with *how* it comes than *when* it comes. As a husband you have, we realize, a social interest in the when. This is like pointing to a particular little green apple developing on an apple tree and asking, "When will that particular apple fall off the tree?" The appropriate answer is "When it's ripe." Good farmers wait for the fruit to ripen. Good obstetricians do not "pick green apples." A good obstetrician has been defined as one equipped with a broad rear end and the good sense to sit calmly on it and let nature take its course.

Of course there are medical indications, in rare instances, that warrant interference and necessitate the forcing of labor before nature acts, such as maternal diabetes, severe Rh sensitization, etc., but these are indeed rare. We are not discussing these rare birds but condemning any thought of forcing a normal baby to come for the convenience of the doctor, the parents, the impatient grandparents, or the thoughtlessly cruel neighbors who look at your wife's big abdomen and ask incredulously, "Haven't you had your baby yet?" then anxiously query, "What's wrong?" One experienced natural childbirth mother got tired of friends and relatives phoning every day after she had gone beyond her due date, asking, "Are you still there?" She answered routinely, "No, this is a recording."

It can be especially nerve-racking to you and your wife if the pregnancy has extended beyond that calculated nine-month calendar date, called the "expected date of confinement" or due date. This ancient ridiculously termed date is two weeks too early anyway—it is calculated upon the onset of your wife's last menstrual period, and even if she is one of those rare women who are accurate record keepers (and most of them aren't; they're only guessing), she wasn't pregnant *then* anyway. Ovulation, and therefore conception, occurs about two weeks after menstruation. Because she can tell when she menstruates and can't tell when she ovulates (unless she's keeping a basal temperature record), down through the ages the calculation has been based upon the obvious sign. This sign, even with a record keeper, is not reliable. There's no such animal as a woman who *always* has regular periods. The ovulation doesn't *always* occur exactly two weeks after menstruation, as our Catholic friends who are depending upon the rhythm method know only too well. Sure as you count on it to, it won't.

To further confuse your calculation some stubborn females may not miss their first, or even second, menstrual period when pregnant. We have had one mother who never missed a menstrual period throughout the entire length of pregnancy with three perfectly normal children.

Any doctor who thinks he can feel your wife's abdomen and tell that the baby is "ready" is fooling himself. He will occasionally pull an apple that is too green, a baby that is not developed far enough to survive independent of its mother.

In the last months of pregnancy those aggravating false labor cramps that make your wife uncomfortable do beneficial things to her baby and her cervix in preparation for the moment of birth. When a patient complains that she is having a lot of false labor, we smile peacefully and say, "Isn't that nice. Your uterus is getting your baby ready." The more false labor your wife has, the less real labor she will have, as these contractions are purposeful and beneficial. They soften and thin (efface) the cervix like

146 : HUSBAND-COACHED CHILDBIRTH

kneading a piece of leather to make it more flexible so it will stretch better later. There are also hormones released by the placenta in the terminal stages of pregnancy which soften a hard cervix and prepare it for dilating.

The false labor contractions also benefit the passenger as well as the passage. The intermittent squeezing and releasing of the baby makes the lungs more dilatable in preparation for taking over breathing when the time comes. In the few women who have a contracted bony pelvis and must have a Caesarean section, we still calmly sit and wait for the onset of labor, even though we know in advance that we are going to operate to get the baby. It would be more convenient for us, and the hospital personnel, if we scheduled the operation on a certain day, at a certain time. We refuse. God schedules a birthday, not man. The contractions of real labor tell us the baby is truly ready. This also helps prevent hyaline membrane formation in its lungs. Hyaline membrane occurs more often in babies delivered early and by Caesarean section.

From the social and psychological standpoint we make two fervent pleas to you as a husband. First, get another woman to come and help your wife by doing the housework (washing, cleaning, cooking, grocery shopping, etc.) for the first two weeks after a new baby is brought home. Let your wife give undivided T.L.C. (tender, loving care), as only a mother can, to the baby. Don't let her helper take care of the baby and your wife end up doing all the work. If the helper is your mother or her mother, she will be tempted to take over the baby. They are such tempting cuddly little bundles of helplessness her mother love will be aroused. Also those older women still tend to consider your wife a little girl and consciously or subconsciously think they know more about caring for babies than your wife does. This isn't so, but even if it were, she will learn by doing, not by observing.

The second fervent plea we make is don't, please don't, call the helper to come *until the baby is born.* Why? There is nothing more productive of anxiety than a prospective grandmother hanging around uselessly, waiting for labor to start. They can undo in a few days all the self-confidence that months of training have accomplished. I recall one case of a nearly hysterical patient who related how her visiting mother paced the floor, wailing, "Oh, you poor dear, if I could just go through this for you." Don't condemn her. Remember she didn't have natural childbirth. She may have had unmedicated, unattended childbirth, but she didn't have careful physical and psychological preparation during pregnancy, and she didn't have a carefully trained coach (husband) to guide her every step. No, don't condemn her; just get rid of her for this stage.

Even if she is a perfect angel and exudes calmness and confidence (they're rare!) she also has her own life to lead and you are wasting her time. You do not need her *before* the baby is born, you need her *afterward.* I can remember many distraught new mothers whose helper wouldn't take this advice and came, bag and baggage, on the calendar due date. But babies can't read calendars! The helper sat uselessly for two weeks, used up her vacation time she had allotted to help her daughter, then departed for home and employment just when the baby was born and she was needed.

Tell your helper what you know—the baby will come when it's good and ready and not until. Have her pass this information to her employer and get permission to start her two-week vacation when your wife calls and tells her she's had the baby.

If you have other children a practical suggestion is to make an agreement with a friend or neighbor to have them come over and take over your home as you leave for the hospital with your wife in labor. If this is the middle of the night your friend or friends can simply go to bed in your bed without disturbing the other children's sleep. Don't, as a husband and labor coach, try to dress and deliver the sleepy older children to someone else's house, because we need *you*. When the baby is born, call your female helper, then go home and relieve your accommodating friend and wait for the helper to arrive.

Please notice I specified *female* helper. Males are good labor coaches but make frustrated, pitiful housewives. You may be entertaining martyr-like thoughts of doing the housework yourself. Don't. Go back to your employment as a breadwinner and let a female take over. Seriously, I'd hate to have to wear the shirt you have washed and ironed. And unless you are indeed a rare bird, I would hate to have to eat the food you have planned and prepared and I have a sneaky feeling your family is in complete agreement with me, even if they wouldn't hurt your feelings by telling you so.

Now, having planned a definite course of action for any conceivable day, or time of day, that your wife may go into real labor, let's explore the question again of when this will happen.

The length of pregnancy in any animal species if each case were plotted on a graph would result in a bell-shaped curve of normal incidence. For instance, let's plot a graph for, say, all the seven-pound babies born in your state for one year. Of course we mean the normal ones allowed to go to spontaneous labor.

The vertical arm of the graph would represent the number of babies, the horizontal arm the months of pregnancy. No matter where you lived on earth the curve would come out the same, bell-shaped. (See graph.)

This typical bell-shaped curve would result also if you similarly plotted the ripening of apples on a tree. A few would ripen early, a few late, and the majority would cluster around the central part of the curve. I thought of this same curve the other night while popping popcorn for the family. My exasperated wife says I see natural childbirth principles in everything! All the popcorn kernels do not suddenly explode simultaneously with a single loud pop. Some start early, then more and more in a crescendo, then the number begins diminishing, with that last slowpoke kernel unexpectedly popping just as you go to pour the corn out, scattering kernels all over the kitchen.

Human babies follow the same pattern. Aggravating as it may be, that's the way it is, has been, and ever shall be with all of nature. There aren't very many seven-pound babies born at six months. The law of the perversity of nature usually takes over so that when one is, the mother got pregnant shortly after marriage, and how the neighbors' tongues wag. It would be as hard to

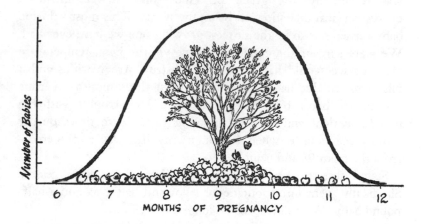

convince them of this rare phenomenon as it was for me to convince a young sailor husband who got his wife pregnant on leave just before sailing overseas. The law of the perversity of nature manifested itself again, as this baby turned out to be one of those slow ones, far beyond the due date. Wouldn't you know!

I had to deal via the Red Cross with a distraught husband overseas, who bitterly claimed "that couldn't be my kid," and a completely hysterical wife who was equally sure it couldn't be anyone else's.

At which point along the curve will *this* particular baby of yours be placed? Who knows?

In healthy normal mothers with healthy normal babies there is no such thing as overdue. This term carries a dire connotation that unjustly scares the daylights out of uninformed people.

More women have been unnecessarily forced into long, hard, unprepared labor, more babies damaged by being made to come through a tough, "green" unripe cervix, because everyone was ready except the baby. It takes an obstetrician with a firm backbone to withstand the onslaught from anxious relatives—"Why don't you *do* something? She's overdue!"

I recall a couple whose long-standing problem of infertility was solved by the grace of God and basal temperature charts, cervical dilatation—in brief, the works. This most valuable baby turned out to be the slowest growing one we have ever had. We were sure of the conception time via the basal temperature chart or we would have assumed menstrual irregularities and a miscalculated due date. The mother went three months overdue and carried her baby a full year. We had no trouble with the grateful patient and her husband, but there were times during those three months when I thought my life was endangered—from the relatives and neighbors!

Sound obstetrical principles we will alter for no social reason. She finally went into spontaneous labor and had a six-and-a-half-pound baby. Why did it wait so long? I don't know.

If your wife goes beyond her due date, don't worry about it. Do take her out more often to be with friends. Get her mind off herself and her baby by distracting her with interesting things to do, interesting people to meet, interesting places to go. Remind her, gently, the baby will come when it is ready.

How to Recognize Real Labor

This sometimes takes a bit of doing, especially if your wife has had previous children. First, let's reassure both of you: There is no such thing as a woman in real labor who doesn't know she's in real labor. It's pretty hard to ignore. If you know perfectly well it's real labor, get to the hospital. Some doctors want to be called first before you leave, others don't. Find out this little detail during your pregnancy. My associates and I are the variety who plead: "If you *know* it's real labor—don't call, get to the hospital."

The reason we don't want our patients to phone if they know they are in real labor is for their own benefit. If the phone call comes in during the night, our telephone secretary may have to reply, "The doctor is tied up in the delivery room now. I'll have him call you when he's free." So the couple sit at home, labor getting harder and harder, waiting for the return call. As they sit and wait I've often wondered just what they expect the doctor to say when he calls. I've often been tempted when a patient says on the phone, "I'm in hard labor, what'll I do?" to answer, "Well, you *could* take in a movie, you *could* visit friends, you *could* go shopping, but then perhaps it would be a better idea to come to the hospital if you know you're going to have a baby!" We do not yield to temptation but simply say, "Come to the hospital." If they had minded our rule in the first place, this delay would not have occurred. While we were finishing up the other case she could have been prepped by the nurse before the labor became so advanced. Don't postpone this preliminary prepping until advanced labor by practicing relaxation at home. Relaxation makes rapid progressive dilatation of the cervix—practice this at the hospital.

I recall one exasperated husband who made a great contribution to our efficiency by asking us why in hades we hadn't given his wife that long complicated hospital admission form for him to fill out during her many office visits? He could have filled it out leisurely at home and had her bring it back. Good idea! That's what we now do. He was exasperated because he missed the birth and very much wanted to be there. He was downstairs filling out the form when she gave birth shortly after arriving. As it turned out it was their own fault this occurred. She had had three previous babies, long, hard labors, and frankly they didn't believe the principles of natural childbirth one bit. They had decided to try it only because "nothing could be worse" than what she had experienced before. When labor had started at home they decided to experiment with it at home to see if it made any difference to relax, breathe with the abdomen, etc. May I make the plea again, don't do this. For two reasons. One, if you wish to experiment, that's perfectly all right but do it in the hospital under the critical eye of the doctor; it's more efficient. Two, you're taking unnecessary chances of not making it to the hospital.

This couple "tried out" the principles at home and barely made it.

Start for the hospital as soon as your wife is convinced that she is in actual labor, for another reason—so you can drive carefully and not have to hurry. Under no, repeat, NO conditions should you exceed the speed limit, run through red lights, or otherwise take silly chances driving. Some frantic, untrained husband ran through a red light in our city and killed two occupants of another car, and his wife had the baby the next day. Police rightly take a dim view of disobeying traffic laws because your wife is in labor. Should the rare occurrence happen that your wife has the baby in the car—let her, and *you* keep driving calmly to the hospital. What do you do with the baby? Nothing. Keep your dirty hands off it and let the doctor or nurse, who is in constant attendance at the emergency room entrance, take care of the baby. Errors committed are always errors of commission, not errors of omission. Your wife can pick it up and put it to her breast and cuddle it if she wishes, should the trip be rather long, but *you* do not need to cut or tie the cord, or try to deliver the placenta, or do anything else except be a chauffeur. These babies and mothers do beautifully, remember. Doctors are necessary when babies won't come, not when they so readily do. All husbands think this might happen to them, but let me reassure you it rarely does. It has happened only three times in my medical career and wouldn't have then if the parents had obeyed the simple rules. It is annoying how often the late ones are parents who live only a few blocks away from the hospital, yet the ones who live at a great distance get there in time.

I recall one hilarious scene at the emergency room entrance as the nurse and I attended such an occurrence. The natural childbirth experienced mother was sitting, tailor fashion, in the back seat of the car in her gown. She was holding the baby to her breast, the umbilical cord intact, the placenta still in place. Her eyes were bright with merriment as she looked at the baby and exclaimed, "Look, isn't he cute?" Then she broke into peals of laughter at her husband's discomfiture. We knew they lived nearby and found out that labor had started two hours before. Why hadn't they started sooner? The mother answered brightly, "I was watching a murder mystery on TV and I waited to see 'who dun it'!"

There are certain handicaps in teaching the self-confidence of natural childbirth to mothers. One of our R.N. teachers, Rhondda Hartman, strolled in calmly with her most recent baby, the third, just ready to be born. Why hadn't she come sooner? we asked. The nonchalant answer was, "I was busy. The La Leche League meeting was at my house tonight." She had calmly finished her job as hostess first, and then, oh, yes, dropped by to have the baby. Her other two children think babies are born at home. She has tucked them in, had the other babies during the night, and gone back home two hours after each birth to greet them in the morning with the new baby. She, like the other teachers, practices what she preaches.

There is no problem, then, if your wife knows she is in labor. Simply come to the hospital.

Now, what if your wife doesn't *know*, just suspects or thinks maybe? Feel free to call your doctor and discuss it with him. Obstetricians don't mind being called at odd hours or they wouldn't be obstetricians. The rewards are magnificent but the hours are terrible!

Before you call the doctor you might try a little test to see if she's in real labor. First, what *is* real labor? Sometimes to be sure it's real labor it takes an examination to see if the cervix is dilating, but there are certain criteria that should tell you without this:

(1) *The uterine contractions should be regular and less than ten minutes apart.* False labor contractions are notable for their irregularity. I remember in my early days of practice I told the class the contractions should be ten minutes apart and forgot to say "or less." As a result a first baby's mother's contractions started two minutes apart and she nearly had the baby at home patiently waiting for them to get to ten minutes apart.

Some labors begin with far-apart contractions, some with close-together ones. The only thing we are sure of, as doctors, is that they are all different. No two labors are exactly alike, even with the same mother. This has been objectively demonstrated by recordings from a tensionometer, a gadget that makes graphs of the uterine muscle activity. In thousands of graphs no two were exactly alike. If your wife has had previous babies, try to persuade her not to judge by what happened last time and expect it to be the same this time. It isn't necessarily so. It may be very different this time.

If her uterine contractions are coming ten minutes apart *or less,* in their regularity, then do they meet the next requirement: (2) Are they progressively harder? Are they picking up and getting stronger? Ask her. Some episodes of false labor have mild contractions which may be less than ten minutes apart. If you apply the tests below, these false contractions will usually fade out and quit. But if her contractions meet these requirements, get her to the hospital without further delay.

If there is doubt in your mind or hers, then you have time to apply the following tests. If the questionable labor began while your wife was up and around, have her do the pelvic rock (horizontal variety) exercise for awhile and then lie down in the side position, curled up in a ball, as previously described. If the questionable labor began during the night while she was reclining or sleeping, have her get up and walk about for a while. In other words, change her activity to the opposite of what she was doing.

If it was only false labor the effect of this change will be to make the contractions less strong, farther apart, and more irregular. Get out your watch and time them (from the start of one to the start of another) before and after the change. If they are farther apart and she feels that they are not as strong, wait awhile and see what happens. They may increase later or they may completely fizzle out.

If this change of activity does *not* affect them and they continue to get more regular, closer, and progressively harder, come to the hospital.

Sometimes that old law of the perversity of nature and women catches up with us. Your wife may meet the test fully at home, and yet the uterine activity may stop after she gets to the hospital.

For reasons which aren't too clear to me this seems to upset the parents. They act embarrassed and apologize profusely to the doctor or nurse for having bothered them. Let me assure you false labor doesn't bother the baby, the doctor, or the nurses. Don't let it bother you if it should happen.

Please take notice I haven't mentioned two phenomena as being part of the indication of true labor. Some patients have the preconceived notion that the water has to break before true labor begins. This is most assuredly not so; some babies are "born with the veil" as it was called in olden times. The water may never break. The baby is pushed out still contained in its intact bag of waters. (I believe superstition has it that babies so born are destined to be great leaders.) Usually the water bag doesn't break until late in labor.

But if it does break at home, and believe me you'll know this if it happens, bring your wife to the hospital, or if it's during regular hours some doctors prefer that you stop at the office. If the water has appeared in a large amount it doesn't matter whether your wife is having uterine contractions or not or what nature they may be—come anyway.

Why? You're more likely to remember to do something if you know why, our principles of natural childbirth dictate. Here's why:

1. The umbilical cord may come down and out with the water. If this happens the presenting part of the baby will put pressure on the cord and compromise the baby's life line. The doctor or nurse wants to listen to your baby's heartbeat (this gives a clue) or check the cervix to tell by feeling if the cord came down. He'll know what to do if this rare thing occurs.

2. She's liable to start hard labor shortly. A few stubborn females don't have labor shortly after the water breaks, but most do. It is noted for being hard, fast, and effective on most occasions. Or putting it another way, you'll probably have to go to the hospital shortly anyway, so you might as well start right away. Get a bath towel to catch the flow of salt water. Sanitary napkins are too small. The salt water comes in intermittent gushes, and some gushes can be quite profuse.

Some mothers are suspicious that their water may have broken but are not sure. This confusion arises from liquefied mucous plugs of the cervix suddenly letting go, and by a tendency in late pregnancy, after the baby has "dropped," to have slight involuntary leakage of urine. These slow leaks are a nuisance but do not yield anywhere near the quantity of fluid present when the water bag really gives way.

This very seldom happens prior to labor, let me repeat. We are amazed that it doesn't happen more often, when you consider how thin and fragile-looking the amniotic sac is and how powerful the uterine muscles are.

The second phenomenon that does *not* have to happen to be true labor is the appearance of blood in the vaginal secretions. We have had patients get this preconceived notion from their grandmother, or some equally unreliable source, and sit at home trying to ignore progressively hard uterine contractions because they couldn't believe it was real labor as they hadn't had a bloody show, as it is called. Bleeding isn't necessary. Its absence does not mean it's not labor, nor does its presence necessarily mean it is labor. All this little dab of bleeding means to a doctor is that the woman is pregnant, and probably has been pregnant before.

Heavy bleeding, as much as a menstrual flow, is a definite abnormality and should be reported to your doctor at once.

The little bloody "spotting" we are discussing comes from the stretching or thinning of the cervix from the effect of false labor. There is much more likelihood of little spots of blood accompanying this if the cervix has previously been stretched with a baby's passage. It can happen occasionally even with the first baby. It usually happens in the last month especially in multiparas (women who have had previous babies), but can happen any time in the last three months. It is caused by the false labor or Braxton Hicks contractions working on the cervix to prepare it for dilatation. It does *not* necessarily mean that the baby is coming early or soon. It is a most unreliable sign of anything, except pregnancy in the last three months.

Backache or lower abdominal cramps are also an unreliable sign of labor. Some labors, depending on the position and size of the baby, have very little backache involved—it's all in front. And vice versa, again depending on the position and size of the baby, the ache may be all in the back, and very little in the front. Pay attention to the original requirements of uterine contractions as listed. Feel the uterus, see what it is doing, time it, ask your wife if it is progressively contracting harder—these indications are reliable.

A Trip Through the Hospital—in Advance

This isn't necessary, it is just nice. If your hospital has a conducted tour to acquaint you with the facilities, avail yourself of it, both you and your wife. Become familiar with which door you enter, especially after daylight hours. Get an admission form beforehand and have it all filled out in advance. Take the tour through the delivery room section. Have the unfamiliar-looking paraphernalia shown and explained to you in advance. Take the tour through the labor room section. Become familiar with the place so that when you arrive with your wife in labor you won't wander aimlessly around, wondering where to go.

Probably the most important thing you can do to keep your wife calm and peaceful as she enters labor is make prior arrangements for the financial coverage of her stay. Hospital admissions offices will have very little sympathy for husbands who had nine long months to make financial arrangements for their wives, then pull that stupid "emergency" idea when their wives go into labor. I've seen perfectly prepared mothers break down in embarrassment and all their preparation go to nought because their husbands had to argue with the admissions office to get them in.

Make financial arrangements, *in advance*. This does not mean you have to have the entire sum of expected expenses as an advance deposit. Hospitals do have credit departments, they do have rules, and they are efficient. They are members of retail credit organizations who keep careful track of all dead beats in their community. If you have a good credit reputation they will honor you.

If you have hospitalization insurance (and in these days you'd have to be a millionaire or a fool not to), bring your policy, visit the admissions office as early as possible during your wife's pregnancy, and make all arrangements. I can't think of a better way to honor the woman you love than to give her the secure feeling you are taking care of her in every way.

There are multiple advantages of unmedicated natural childbirth. One of these, you will discover to your pleasure, is less hospital expense. There is no anesthetist fee when there is no anesthetist. Also the comparatively short stay of unmedicated mothers and babies can reduce the bill. Neither mother nor baby is "sick" and their stay can be shortened. (See Chapter 10.)

"If We Have a Boy, Should He Be Circumcised?"

This will apply to half the readers, but no one knows in advance which half. Most doctors feel newborn boys should be circumcised before leaving the hospital. Why?

The foreskin serves no useful purpose in humans. In the four-legged animals it probably serves to protect the more sensitive end of the penis (glans) from bruising and scratching while running on all fours through brush and bramble.

It can be a source of much trouble in humans. Unless bathed and cleansed daily, bacteria get in the mucous-like secretion which accumulates underneath it. I doubt that many boy babies actually *have* to be circumcised due to tightness and elongation of the foreskin (phimosis). However, in nearly all babies the retraction of this skin in order to cleanse away the secretion underneath is usually not easily accomplished by the new mother. If she manages to get it retracted it is sometimes so tight a fit that swelling occurs and she can't get it back down again. All of this operation is usually accompanied by the indignant shrieking of the baby, which upsets an already nervous new mother.

As the child gets older he must learn to keep up the daily bathing or accept the risk of infection.

During my tour of duty as a navy doctor the naval hospital wards were being constantly cluttered with grown men convalescing from circumcisions. This high incidence of needed circumcisions in the sailors during the war could have been related to the interference with regular bathing during battle conditions. Judging by the comments and vivid poetry written by these men regarding the recovery phase, the adult age is the tender age to have this done. Swelling and pain is terrific in older age groups and healing proportionately slow.

Newborn babies pay little attention and need no anesthetics. Because of the small size at this age an efficient clamp seals the edges of the cut skin so stitches aren't necessary. Healing is rapid and apparently pain-free—in newborns. Mothers need to take a lot of care of an uncircumcised baby's penis, but no particular care of the circumcised one.

Should infection ensue later in the uncircumcised, or the mother be unable to replace the retracted foreskin, the proper treatment is circumcision. Later, after the baby has grown, he would need an anesthetic and stitches, and would have a longer and more painful recovery period. The advocates for circumcision feel prevention is better than cure.

There is a psychological indication too for circumcising your boy. A generation ago any circumcised boy swimming nude at the YMCA was probably of Jewish descent and in the minority. The wisdom of the Jewish leaders has now become so widely accepted that there is a complete turnabout. The uncircumcised boy is the rarity and by looking different is subject to the thoughtless cruelty of scorn from playmates. Children can be unthinkingly cruel.

It is so simple to circumcise the baby before he is taken home, and it saves the mother and the child a lot of trouble later. Assume you're going to have a boy and make up your mind before you have the baby, so you will be prepared to sign the permit if you wish upon entering the hospital. A circumcision permit is part of the admission form.

10

Postpartum and Family Relations

AFTER HAVING THE BABY and drinking the iced orange juice "honorary cocktail" given as a reward to natural childbirth parents, the next question we hear from both parents is "When can I go home? or "When can she go home?" Our usual answer is, "You just got here. Why talk about going home?"

How long should your wife stay in the hospital? The answer to that is, as long as she wishes. How long should the baby stay in the hospital? The answer here is, barring prematurity or complications, As short a time as possible. Why? As Dr. Thaddeus Montgomery has stated, "The hospital is a good place to deliver a baby but a poor place to board it."[1] If your hospital is modern enough to have rooming-in facilities, the only hurry to get the baby out would be financial. The rent comes high. If they don't have rooming-in facilities, then get the baby home as soon as possible. What's the hurry? Because of the mixing of bacteria from other babies by putting them all in a large nursery together. I care not how "sterile" the technique, this is bacteriologically ridiculous. Babies don't get infections from themselves or their mothers (they are born with acquired immunity to the mother's bacteria); they get them from other babies. Also babies cannot read hospital feeding schedules. They want to eat on their own schedule and this very rarely happens to coincide with the nurs-

[1] Montgomery, T. L.: Amer. J. Obst & Gyn 81: 890-901, 1961.

161

ery's schedule—as evidenced by their frustrated crying. Besides, for psychological reasons babies should stay with their mothers. The best person to care for the baby is its mother. The nurses may be the best nurses available, but they are not *the* mother. And don't think that baby of yours doesn't notice the difference. Later on he must be temporarily separated from his mother, for a few hours each week, to find out there are others. But the first two weeks of life, especially the first few hours and days, represents an extreme change in his life to which he must adjust.

Imagine for a while the nature of the changes in his world that occurred at birth. From 98.6-degree warmth to 70-degree room temperature. From total darkness to glaring overhead lights in the hospital. From relative quiet where instead of mother's familiar voice and the soothing rhythmical sounds of her body (her heartbeat, breath sounds, etc.) there are sudden loud, unfamiliar, startling noises. From being carried constantly with the rocking motion from mother's hip movements, to the utter stillness of a crib. From soft smooth salt water feelings to dry sterile harsh sheets (you will see red rash on the baby's skin from contact). From being fed continuously from mother's body via the life line, to being ignored until it's convenient for the nurses. Can you blame any baby for wanting to go home with mother? For wanting to be loved, and held, and rocked, and talked to, and fed when hungry?

Now, what about the mother? Actually she needs rest the first few hours. But have you ever been around a hospital long? She will rest far better in her own familiar bed at home, hearing the familiar noises she is so accustomed to, as opposed to clanging bed pans, squawking call systems, talking personnel, patients and visitors. For goodness' sake, take her home. Remember to have the helper there to do the work; with this arrangement most mothers would much rather be home.

Unmedicated mothers and unmedicated normal-sized babies are not sick and do far better at home. The average stay for natural childbirth patients in our hospital is twenty-four hours. A few of our athletes insist on going immediately after the two-hour period of observation following the birth. In the absence of medication or complication we have always allowed this—if they are breast feeding. We know the nursing will keep the postpartum uterus tight.

After arriving home there will be a period of adjustment for the husband. The "little stranger," as grandmother called the baby, can surely disrupt the interpersonal relationship between you and your wife—as you remembered it. She hardly ever has time for you. She will later, so don't let it throw you. She was such a good housekeeper before! Now look at the place! Hold your horses, she will be neat again—later. There just isn't time enough when the baby is so little. Don't be demanding and expect exotic meals to be prepared this time. Rather, ask if you can't bring home some prepared food to relieve her duties. And don't expect your meals right on time as they used to be—baby takes precedence. Later on things will get back to schedule, so cheer up!

Love-making? She can't be bothered with it now, psychologically or physically. Wait—for about six weeks. After her postpartum check at six weeks the doctor will plan with her the method of choice for spacing her pregnancies if she so desires. Babies are bundles of joy, but not when they come every nine months!

Well, what can *you* do? In the midst of all this female activity you may feel a little lost and left out, and definitely ignored on occasions. Rest assured that just your presence makes a great difference. She knows you're around. You ought to see the nervous wrecks of mothers who don't have husbands to bring them home!

What happened to your role as a coach? It's still there. Let's review some of the things you can coach and remind your wife to do now, as you did during pregnancy and labor.

Physical Factors

Your wife's three "B" muscles (back, belly, bottom) have done their duty, but they have been necessarily stretched and weakened from use. They need to be strengthened and tightened to restore her to the nonpregnant shape. The postpartum exercises are nearly identical to the prepartum, with the addition of more vigorous abdominal exercises. There was no point during pregnancy of trying to draw in abdominal muscles that were steadily going out.

Again, the ancient idea that your wife can't take a bath has been shown to be ridiculous. After about three days she should take a long, hot, leisurely bath twice a day for two weeks, then daily. The penetrating heat of soaking a part of your body is more beneficial and effective than surface heat. In most hospitals they still use heat lamps on her bottom. We far prefer hot tub baths. If you have a sore thumb you don't shine a light on it, you soak it in hot water to reduce the swelling and increase the rate of healing by increased circulation. The same goes here after having a baby. After about three days she should wear internal tampons (large size) to absorb the lochial drainage which is normal for about a month following the birth. If she goes out in public for long periods she should wear *both* the internal protection and the external pads because the discharge may come in irregular amounts and it's hard to tell when the internal tampon is saturated. A sanitary napkin will allow her to enjoy the church service without worry. At home there is no need for external pads. External napkins can cause irritation and possible infection. At home if she feels moisture coming around the internal tampon, she merely stops her activity to go change. These internal tampons can be left in while taking the tub bath. If she had stitches, don't worry about it. The tampons absorb the moisture before it gets down to the level of the stitches and prevents infection from developing. The heat of the bath reduces swelling and promotes healing of the incision as well as providing a cleansing action.

The external vaginal skin needs protection from moisture and infection. Bathing this area should be done with soap substitutes containing hexachlorophene, just as before the baby. We further suggest that she use the same oil preparation on herself that she uses on her baby. The same application is suggested for the same reason, to prevent diaper rash in the baby, and to prevent panty rash in the mother. If she really wants healthy skin in this area, she should abstain from panties *for life*.

She should continue the same vitamin and iron supplementary pills that were prescribed during pregnancy, at least until the doctor checks her at six weeks and as long as she continues to breast feed. Some doctors prescribe additional iron pills in the postpartum period to compensate for the necessary blood loss following normal births.

Exercises

These are essentially a repetition of the prenatal ones, like tailor sitting and squatting in her work. Now with a new baby she will have additional work that can utilize these beneficial exercises. Baby's diapers should be changed *on the floor*. She should put an extra baby blanket on the floor and squat or tailor sit while supporting the baby in one arm. She can change the diaper and put the baby back under her arm—hillbilly style—with his head held in the palm of her hand, his wiggly legs securely wedged between her upper arm and her chest, his back properly supported on her forearm, and then rise "tail first," just as before.

One of our patient's mothers criticized her daughter for carrying her new baby around like that—"You look like a hillbilly!" Don't argue with your mother, but don't pay any attention either —she doesn't know. The two-armed method is O.K. when you and your wife are sitting down rocking the baby, but it is dangerous when walking. The one-armed method is safe, as the baby can't suddenly draw his feet back and lurch out of your arms when your attention is diverted.

Also if you should trip or step on a roller skate unexpectedly and fall while you are carrying the baby with both arms, he will go sailing across the room. The reflex of self-preservation automatically takes over and your arms fly out to catch yourself, temporarily forgetting about the baby.

Your wife won't need to do any extra tailor sitting or squatting; just taking care of the baby will give her plenty of opportunity.

Sitting on a hard floor, even if carpeted, sounds uncomfortable if your wife had stitches, but it only sounds that way. Actually she will be more uncomfortable sitting a soft seat. Why? Because on the firm floor she sits down on her sitting-down bones (ischial tuberosities) and these aren't sore, as the stitches aren't near them. The stitches are in the flesh up between these bony prominences, and the floor doesn't hit the sensitive area as a cushion or soft seat would.

The pelvic rocking you should insist on before allowing her in bed at night—for the rest of her life. Professional models, movie stars, and others do this to keep their bodies and posture beautiful. Your wife's body is just as important. If "after pains" become a nuisance at home, she should pelvic rock and curl up on her side at intervals during the day. She will not only look better, she will feel better.

The "running" position of sleep—on her side with top leg pulled up, is equally applicable for the rest of her life after having the baby! In the immediate postpartum it seems to allow the still heavy uterus to fall freely forward, which is important in preventing a backward or "tipped" uterus from developing.

The exercise for the Kegel (vaginal, bladder, and rectal) muscle should be continued as during the pregnancy (see Chapter 6 for review). A good additional time to perform it is while she is nursing or feeding the baby. Ask her if she's doing it and remind her to.

The abdominal muscles need the most attention, as they were stretched the most over the longest period of time. Most hospitals furnish directional diagrams on how to perform these, or, even better, she may learn them by attending a postpartum exercise class. The time for performing extra or deliberate abdominal muscle exercises is on awakening. It took nine months to stretch those muscles, remember, and it takes nine months to tighten them. Accordingly, set your alarm clock ten minutes earlier for the next nine months after the baby comes and get your wife to do these deliberate abdominal muscle calisthenics every morning during this period. If you're an office worker, may I make a suggestion? Do them with her. It won't hurt you to have a flat stomach too!

After two weeks of continuous T.L.C. (tender, loving care) of the baby, get a baby sitter and take your wife out once a week, for the rest of your lives together, for some sport that involves great vigor. Swimming is ideal (she can insert a fresh tampon, large size, just before entering the pool). Golf, tennis, square dancing, bowling—it doesn't matter which. What did you do before she had a baby? Do it again, and do it regularly. Social exercises, participating with a group of friends, are not only more fun but more likely to be regularly pursued. Calisthenics at home get boring.

How much activity should your wife have after having a baby? Whatever she feels like. Just as during pregnancy, she will tire more rapidly. Having a baby is hard work and she has donated a portion of her reserve energy to her baby—that's where he got it. Her reserves will gradually build up. They will build up more rapidly if she returns to her usual type of conduct. Again, she may not be able to swim as many laps, bowl as many games, etc., as before her pregnancy. This does not mean she shouldn't indulge and should become a sedentary figure. It means she should stop and rest when she tires. Let her decide.

There is a silly superstition that she shouldn't go up and down steps after having a baby. She shouldn't *have to* go up and down steps constantly in her work. To try to get things she *has* to do on the same level would be very helpful in her work. But she can go up and down steps if she takes her time about it and doesn't overtire herself.

Another silly superstition is that women can't drive cars after having babies. If she is an experienced driver there is no earthly reason why not. In fact she should have a car available for her own use, if it is financially feasible, now that she has a baby. Her household supplies may run out and she needs to shop more often to meet the baby's needs. Also she shouldn't feel tied down so she can't go anywhere. She will tend to blame this tied-down feeling on the baby, when it's just lack of transportation. And babies love to ride in cars. The older and more rickety the car, the more it vibrates and rattles, the more they like it. If you want to soothe a colicky, fussy baby, take it for a ride in the car. The rhythmical vibrations of the motor tend to soothe it.

Psychological "Togetherness"

All parents have misgivings about their capabilities of parenthood. These are magnified by reading the confusing multitude of books advising parents. Limit this reading to avoid confusions. I would suggest two books as being perfectly adequate for ready reference on any problems that may arise: *The Family Book of Child Care* by Dr. Niles Newton and *The Pocket Book of Baby and Child Care* by Dr. Benjamin Spock. Consult your doctor or pediatrician about anything that can't be cleared up by the advice in these books.

If this is your first baby, remember the old saying: Babies grow up in spite of the parents, not due to them. Your only real responsibility is to "have 'em, love 'em, and leave 'em be." Let them be little individuals. Don't try to force your preconceived notions of what you think they ought to do or be upon them as they grow. Let them be themselves, and take joy in the privilege of being with them for a while. In the steadily increasing life span of both of you, the period during which children are dependent upon you is, proportionately, very short. Enjoy it. They begin to acquire independence surprisingly early. They need guidance and chaperoning, of course, but don't try to make a round peg fit in a square hole. Let them be what they are, not what you think they ought to be.

Get a baby sitter once a week, beginning when the baby is two weeks old, and let someone else take him over for a few hours. Now of course pick some mature, kindly person you can depend on to exercise good judgment and common sense, but get the idea out of your head that you and your wife are the only ones who can take care of your children! Such egotism is unwarranted.

Grandmother says, "You had them and you should never leave them." Such martyrdom is selfish and harmful to both you and the child. Someday such clinging, dependent children will have to be torn from their mothers and get the rude shock that there are other people in the world—on the first day at school, for instance. This shock will be far less and the adjustment to the presence of other residents of this planet far better if they get a sneak preview in advance that there are others. There is nothing more sickening to see than a child throwing a tantrum ("Don't leave me, don't leave me!") when the parents are going out for an evening. If they have been regularly introduced to baby sitters since they were two weeks old, they are intellectually curious about outsiders. They get sick and tired of looking at their parents constantly and will tend to ask later, "Don't you two ever go anywhere?" They will accept and like the challenge of meeting strangers. Also parents tend to get tired of their children ("They get on my nerves!") if they are never separated for regular short intervals.

Clinging children grow up to be clinging adults. There is no more pitifully inadequate father or husband than a "mama's boy." The same inadequacy holds for a "mama's girl." They are frightened to be on their own and have to run back to mamma for advice—even as adults. Such misfits are made by subconscious selfishness on the part of parents who feel their children should feel an indebtedness for just being born. Be proud of your children's independence, be ashamed of clinging dependence. Dr. Edward A. Strecker's books *Their Mothers' Sons*[2] and *Their Mothers' Daughters*[3] should be read by both of you after your children get older.

Parents who foster feelings of indebtedness and overdependency in their children are reflecting their own sense of inadequacy. Be someone in your own right and let your children do likewise. They will admire and respect you in adulthood as they loved you in childhood.

That most horrible of monsters, the All-American "Mom," has been derided by the famous author Philip Wylie many times in many ways. I was delighted to read in the *Reader's Digest* the preview of his daughter's book, *Nursing Your Baby*,[4] by Karen Pryor, on the La Leche League and breast feeding. She certainly doesn't sound like a selfish, pay-me-back kind of mom.

Parents who keep their children clingingly dependent on them also keep themselves clingingly dependent on their children. In the animal kingdom one doesn't see parents closely following their children to "help" them after the children achieve adult stature.

Natural childbirth trained parents are noted for the low incidence of divorce. The main cause of the breakup of young couples that I have seen in my office has been meddlesome parents who patly rationalize that they are only "helping" their son or daughter. They are so dependent upon their children that they have lost all their own individuality and become complete bores, particularly to themselves. The further unfortunate thing, for their children, is that they will live forever—or so it will seem to their children. The life expectancy is steadily rising, and old age pensions are steadily rising along with it. Soon there will be a

[2] J. B. Lippincott, Philadelphia, 1961.
[3] J. B. Lippincott, Philadelphia, 1956.
[4] Harper & Row, New York, 1963.

little handful of slaving young people burdened with the huge taxation that doles out financial reward and sustenance for a huge army of idle, usless old people, whining to their children, "I gave birth to you, pay me back!" Add to this the likelihood that your wife will outlive you and see the picture.

Am I building up to the idea that a "young-age pension" would be more logical? No, I want you, and especially your wife, not to get so involved with your children that you have nothing else to think about or talk about. What utter bores such people are. Continue while the children are young some line of intellectual pursuit which will stand you in good stead when they are grown and gone—and don't you dare tag along "helping" them. Have 'em, love 'em, and leave 'em be! In order to do the latter let your wife continue her education via the many wonderful opportunities for adult education or Continuation Study Centers available now. You might study some together, even though as a husband you have your work which will stand you in good stead a good deal of your life. If all she has is children, they will not be needing her in a few years; and if she has maintained no other interest there is a great letdown. There is a psychological feeling of having outlived her usefulness that makes the menopause a period of great depression. Her life should truly *begin* at forty if She has something left after having done her duty to her children. She should be so busy with her own interests then that she doesn't have time for adult children. Help her keep those interests up when her children are little. Don't make a drudge out of her. This can be prevented by letting her have one evening or afternoon to herself in school or a career while the children are young. When the last youngster enters school full time, so should she—or pursue a career she loves.

Housework and children are rewarding too, but they should not be allowed to be so all-encompassing that she loses her individuality. Do you want to be leading a cow down the road of life, or trying to keep step with a race horse?

11

The Husband's Role in Breast Feeding

W<small>E HAVE TAKEN NOTE</small> of the Carnation Milk Company's famous slogan that contented cows give better milk. Nervousness interferes with milk formation in human mothers too. We have finally found the main cause of nervousness in women—men.

We have also found the main cause of contentment in women —educated, understanding men.

As specialists in teaching women childbirth without fear (natural childbirth) we have found the cooperation of husbands indispensable. Statistics illustrate the importance of togetherness at this time. Both obstetricians who forbid the participation of the husband and hospitals which exclude him from the delivery room have more anxious, frightened mothers who plead for medication and require more forceps deliveries than if they had received no prenatal instruction at all.

The same holds for breast feeding. The success or failure of breast feeding depends primarily on the attitude of the husband toward it. His attitude will depend, in turn, upon experiences in his past, even early childhood, in relationship to breast feeding.

I recall one young couple on their first visit in the office, in the wife's first pregnancy. I asked the wife if she planned to breast feed her baby. She never had a chance to answer. The husband shot out of his chair and declared in a hostile tone, "She is not." I looked surprised and asked why not. "I married her because of her breasts, they're mine, and I'm not going to have any kid touching them, including my own!" He was only expressing openly what a lot of men unknowingly manage to convey in subtle ways to subconsciously discourage their wives.

Could such exaggerated importance of the breasts be related to his frustration from early weaning, or bottle feeding, or perhaps the power of suggestion from every book cover, billboard, and auto tire advertisement? Will he become a Hollywood serial polygamist seeking a younger set of breasts in rotation when one set gets soft and less shapely from age and use? What a basis for marriage!

Let's start from scratch. Why should you subtly or openly *encourage* your wife to nurse her baby? What difference does it make? to whom? Is there some magic in mother's milk? As men we must admit that breasts do make lovely sweater decorations. However, as doctors, we remind you that their primary purpose is a source of food for babies. Any part of the human body is healthier when used properly for its intended purpose. Cancer of the breast occurs less in breasts that have been used to feed babies.

As a doctor, an obstetrician, the benefits we seek are primarily to your wife. Let's consider a few. We think the Creator intended that your wife should not have an immediate return of her menstrual bleeding after having a baby. She has donated blood to the baby itself (not directly but via the ingredients), she then loses some incident to its birth. The recovery phase from this loss after the baby is .born should not be handicapped by menstruation. It's hard to build up a depleted savings account when regular withdrawals are made. The breasts serve as a valve to shut off menstruation by suppressing ovulation after the baby is born. Some women may have menstrual periods while breast feeding (even these are lighter!) but most women do not.

Men hardly ever have "tired blood" or low levels of hemoglobin, but many women do. Prevention is better than the alcoholic elixirs advertised on TV as a cure for "tired blood." Breast feeding mothers have higher blood levels. They are more energetic, feel better, and are more fun to live with and be around.

The uterus contracts by reflex during breast feeding. This causes it to shrink back (involute) faster to its nonpregnant size. This means less backache, pelvic dragging feeling, varicose veins, etc., from a big heavy uterus. If your wife bottle feeds, you're the one who has to live with this droop, remember.

Regardless of what method of baby-spacing you choose, the first to consider is nature's, especially if you're Roman Catholic in faith. It doesn't always work (which one does?), but it definitely postpones fertility after a baby is born. If used in conjunction with other methods, babies can be planned.

Then there is the psychological effect of this "womanly art" on your wife. She is more of a mother in her own eyes and those of her friends. Women who have failed to breast feed will tend to resent her and ridicule the procedure. Could their own slips be showing? Your wife, later on, having gradually weaned her babies from her breast physically will be better able to wean them from her *psychologically* when the time comes. Her children won't suffer from "Mom-ism." She will also be a more calm, kind, considerate person for you to live around. The close physical contact with baby triggers the outflow of true selfless compassion for all humanity. The intermittent peaceful moments during the day when she must sit down and hold her baby give her body rest and her soul peace.

What about the baby? From a strict nutritional standpoint cow's milk can be supplemented with vitamins and additives until it seems to contain all the chemicals necessary for growth. However there's more to it than chemicals. The protein and other ingredients in milk seem to be specific for each species of animal. Cow's milk was designed for calves. Human milk for humans. When the species is crossed, allergic reactions sometimes develop from "foreign" protein ingestion.

Even so, breast-fed babies are known to grow better, have

fewer infections, have less colic, and be more content than the ones on the fanciest cow milk formula yet devised. Why? For psychological reasons.

Let's recall, again, the intrauterine environment where the baby spent nine peaceful dependent months. There were no stresses, no challenges that had to be met, no startling new experiences to have to adjust to. The advent of birth changed all this, as the baby began the first step towards eventual independence.

It's necessary to leave the comforts and serenity of home and go out into the unknown and conquer the dragons. But isn't it nice to come back home again, especially for some of that good old home cooking? Isn't it easier to digest your food in the familiar surroundings of home?

Babies are the same way. After leaving "home" they like to come back, temporarily, for dinner. When a mother holds her baby against the warmth of her skin it reproduces that 98.6-degree body warmth known before. The smooth softness of the breast is similar in touch sensation to the lining of the uterus. Watch the baby fondle and caress the breast during feeding. The fragrance of mother's skin oils is pleasing to his nostrils. Is this how calves so accurately select their own mothers in a herd of similar-looking cows? Perhaps the individual protein content of her milk tells his taste buds he's home again. It's hard to test these particular senses—temperature, touch, and smell—in human babies scientifically and objectively. The importance of temperature and touch in the recognition and acceptance of mother was brilliantly, scientifically demonstrated by the work of Dr. Harry F. Harlow[1] in rhesus monkey experiments at the University of Wisconsin.

After isolating baby monkeys from their real monkey mothers, he offered them cleverly devised substitute "mothers." These surrogate mothers were inanimate and doll-like in nature and of varied color, texture, and temperature.

The two important physical characteristics which made these

[1] "Affectional Responses in the Infant Monkey," *Science*, Aug. 21, 1959, Vol. 130, No. 3373, pp. 421-32.

substitutes acceptable to the baby monkeys were softness to the touch and warmth. The babies would select the warm, soft ones over the others as their choice of mother figures.

Dr. L. Salk,[2] the psychologist brother of the inventor of polio vaccine, Dr. Jonas Salk, used human babies to objectively demonstrate the benefit of one aspect of babies' hearing sense, the mother's heartbeat.

He divided a hospital nursery into two sections and reproduced the recorded sound of a mother's heartbeat over a speaker in one nursery and not in the other, then studied the effect on the babies. He conclusively verified by experimentation an assumption of ours that we have been describing to our patients for years—that human babies, hearing a mother's heartbeat, are more serene, digest their food better, and even grow better than babies who don't hear a mother's heartbeat.

If you obtain a puppy or kitten while it is quite young and separate it from its mother for the first time, it will cry piteously at night. Put two items in its box and the household will be undisturbed—an electric heating pad and a ticking alarm clock! It isn't mother but it seems to do until something better shows up.

Put a cheap, loud-ticking clock in your baby's bedroom and the baby will sleep better. Why? Because during the intrauterine life he become accustomed to the rhythmical sounds of mother's heart beating.

It hasn't been tested, but still another assumption seems reasonable—the rhythmical breath sounds of the mother's lungs, the soft swishing sound heard through a doctor's stethoscope, can also be heard by the baby. We call this the "breeze in the trees" sound as heard at night in the mountain cabin. Don't you sleep like a baby there?

[2] L. Salk: "The effects of the normal heartbeat sound on the behavior of the newborn infant; implications for mental health." *World Mental Health*, 12:168-175, 1960.

During the act of breast feeding, the rhythmical rise and fall of your wife's chest reproduces for your baby a motion sense similar to that caused by her abdominal breathing during sleep, when your baby was in her uterus. Let's add another motion familiar to a baby—rocking. A keen observer can notice the pregnant state of a woman by the rocking motion of her hips as she walks by. This is a consequence of the softening of her pelvic joints making them mobile, the effect of hormones from the placenta. This brings up two mother commandments in feeding a newborn. First, she should hold the baby against the warmth of her body. If she is breast feeding, this is inescapable, but should be done even if bottle feeding. Never, never prop a bottle on something, then desert the baby. Second commandment, you should invest in a rocking chair and have her rock the baby while he's feeding or when he's fussy. Let's add a third commandment for your wife— verbalize! Hum, sing, or talk to him in a singsong manner. She doesn't have to be a professional singer, just herself. The baby is used to the sound of her voice—he listened to it for nine months in the uterus. As a doctor, if we are trying to hear the baby's heartbeat through the fetoscope in the prenatal examinations and the mother starts talking, we hastily remove the instrument from our ears; her voice is transmitted so loudly it is uncomfortable.

One theory of why teenagers prefer and enjoy the loud rhythms of rock and roll music is that they are meeting their heaviest challenges at adolescence and like to return temporarily to the security of the womb. As experience produces true self-confidence later, such prominent rhythmic beats will not be necessary. But even lots of mature people like background music and find it restful.

Could it be that being cheated out of these reassuring rhythmical sounds by the predominance of bottle feeding plays a role in the delayed maturing of some adults, like the beatniks?

In summary then, encourage your wife to breast feed your baby. Do this in kind, subtle ways as well as in verbal ones.

Defend her from the attacks of envious females whose criticism comes from their jealousy. If in the rare instance she cannot breast feed for some reason or other, all is not lost. Simply remind her to hold your baby, rock it, caress it, talk or sing to it while it is eating. *How* it is fed is probably far more important than *what* it is fed.

12

The Nature of Instinct

NATURAL CHILDBIRTH CONCEPTS are based upon the principle that human beings are not instinctive animals and must be taught to do what lower animals automatically do without training. As we have stressed before, this difference between human beings and other animals is obvious in their respective conduct in water and in labor.

However, anyone contemplating this theory would reflect on some instances in which human behavior under the stress of childbirth labor or in keeping afloat in water seemed to demonstrate instinctive, automatic behavior—without preliminary training. Indeed, Dr. Grantly Dick-Read was first inspired by the calm instinctive conduct of a mother who smilingly turned down his offer of gas because "God didn't intend it to hurt."

Any medical personnel associated with obstetrics very long will be impressed by the variety of conduct of different women in labor. Not all untrained mothers in labor panic, scream, and ask to be "knocked out" and "delivered." I can use the example of my own six-foot-tall, deeply religious, English-Canadian mother who not only calmly gave unmedicated birth to eleven pounds of me, but kidded the attending doctor because *he* perspired and *she* didn't.

Could it be possible that, after all, human beings *do* have instinctive powers?

Let's consider the human brain and its function and "brain-storm" a bit about this elusive ability known as instinct. Could it possibly be that human brains do share this ability with other animals but that somewhere in the evolutionary development of more complex brains we have lost the ability to use it in most instances?

In the anatomic examination of the human brain we find an "older" portion which resembles that of the lower animals. The outer covering or cortex of the human brain, which presumably evolved more recently, is much thicker and more complex than that of the lower animals. This is the portion which is thought to function in abstract thinking and reasoning. In human beings it is highly developed.

With all this superior equipment, why do we humans have to be "delivered" of our young as if they were something evil and abnormal? Or do we? Not in some instances. Why the difference?

If as a labor coach you are to be effective, you must be convincing. In order to be convincing to your wife you must first be convinced in your own mind. Toward that end let's consider the function of human brains. Brevity dictates oversimplification, but your relationship to your wife and to your child depends upon insight into these functions.

In my opinion human brains do have full instinctive abilities, just like those of the lower animals. For convenience we think of these abilities as being housed and functioning in the inner older "animal" part of our brain. For simplicity we will refer to this area as governing the subconscious.

Why do only *some* human beings under some conditions sometimes manifest instinct? If it's so beneficial, why do not all people use it at all times? Because it is not always available for use. The cortex of human brains can, because of its very complexity, act as a cover-up to the underlying animal brain. This outer layer, for convenience, we will refer to as controlling the conscious mind of man. These two functions are not mutually exclusive, the

conscious and the subconscious. Rather they are constantly interacting and affecting each other. The more complicated the conscious mind has become, the more it interferes with instinctive
abilities.

For instance, prior to the age of six months, human infants
manifest swimming instinct; they either swim automatically or
are very easy to teach. After six months the conscious cover-up
begins to form. Learning responsibility results in development of
fear, anxiety, and worry, which interferes with instinctive
conduct.

Could the religious convictions of my mother and Dr. Dick-
Read's patient have caused a serenity which thinned the clouds
of anxiety and fear, allowing the automatic guidance of instinct
to penetrate? As an obstetrician I have seen this many times.

Can prenatal education and guidance coupled with the reassuring presence of the man she loves, constantly coaching and encouraging, allow your wife to function as an instinctive animal,
enabling her to joyously give birth? Yes, indeed, I have seen this
many, many times too.

Why are some women so much easier to teach to give birth
than others? Let's answer that by substituting for convenience
the instinctive function, swimming, for that of birth. Why are
some human beings so much easier to teach to swim than others?
Could the individual who "takes to water like a duck" possess a
thinner conscious cloud layer than the difficult pupil whose cloud
layer was thickened by fear of water due to some unpleasant
previous experience or, perhaps, fear following gruesome suggestions planted previously by thoughtless people?

Even the most frightened conscious-clouded human being can,
by patient instruction and reassurance, overcome fear and anxiety
and be taught to swim. The same applies to your wife and childbirth. Barring physical abnormalities there is no woman who
can't by patient instruction be taught to give birth.

These are only two manifestations of instinct. To understand
its nature further, what instinctive functions other than swim-

ming and birth might be manifested by human beings? Are these others also applicable to our lives?

Instinct has been recognized for many centuries although the exact nature of it and *how* it works has not as yet been determined. It is about time we quit ignoring the irrefutable fact that it works and turn the academic light of science upon it for a more thorough study. The possibility that human beings may share instinctive abilities with animals has awakened some interest. Increasing evidences that support this possibility are being brought to light. We have much to gain in better interpersonal relations by more extensive studies in this area.

Telepathy falls within the category of human instincts. What does recognizing the telepathic ability of some human beings have to do with your life, your wife, your baby? More than you perhaps realize. Babies and young children have thin conscious-cloud layers due to inexperience and dependence. Their little telepathic receivers function very efficiently. An article in a popular magazine recently featured brain-wave tracing of a mother and her infant taken all night long during sleep. It was observed that the pattern of pleasant dreaming and unpleasant, disturbed dreaming was identical for both mother and child. In other words the baby, even while asleep, sensed each time its mother was disturbed. When its mother was serene, so was the baby. Was this an objective measurement of human instinctual telepathy?

Apply this to other human relationships. What are the practical aspects of awareness of such human communicability? Plenty! Thoughts run through my mind of that young couple who had a baby to "hold their marriage together." They sweet talk each other in front of the child while harboring hostility toward each other in their subconscious "animal" minds—and wonder why the child becomes a nervous, neurotic, insecure individual. He senses that hostility telepathically. Don't try to kid kids!

Another disturbing memory comes to my mind: P.T.A. meetings where I have met frustrated women who are teaching elementary school but who do not like children. Their syrupy sweet talk before the class goes for nought. These children sense that subconscious dislike and react with hostility. How much better children perform and what inspiration they receive when a compassionate woman who truly loves children is guiding them subconsciously.

Clairvoyance is another category of instinct. Is there a "mind's-eye" at this level which can see, even at great distances and in spite of physical obstacles? This is evidenced in animals' homing instinct, the sore-footed cat or dog that returns home no matter where it's taken. Why can't we lose them? They seem to be able to "see" home, even an empty house when no one is there. (If some person or animal is present at home this would complicate the picture by the possibility of its being telepathic perception.) This was dramatically illustrated in Walt Disney's film, *The Incredible Journey*, relating the ability of two dogs and a cat to return to an empty home over great distances and in spite of many obstacles in the path. Can human minds do this? There are many evidences that they can. A high percentage of similar phenomena occur in interpersonal relationships of mother love and other close emotional ties. The mother "sees" the exact scene of an accident involving her child, etc.

Just for fun you and your wife can play a little game testing her subconscious "animal" instinctual ability.

Is she carrying a boy or girl baby? Her logical conscious mind when asked this question would result in only a 50-50 guessing accuracy. However her subconscious animal mind utilizing the sixth sense has a reputation for higher accuracy. How do you eliminate her conscious mind? By applying the ancient pendulum test. In psychological circles this is referred to as ideomotor activity which is muscular action reflecting responses from subconscious mind activity.

Don't depend entirely on the results, but just for fun do repeated tests and check the results. Here's how. Tie any weighted object (traditionally your wedding ring) on a length of thread.

Have your wife hold it over the palm of a man or boy then over the palm of a woman or girl while keeping her *eyes closed.* This is to eliminate her conscious mind from knowing the result. To the best of her ability she should try to hold the thread still. As an observer you will note, however, that the weighted object will go back and forth when held over a male palm and in a circular motion over a female palm. After establishing this with a few test runs, then have your wife lie down, eyes closed, and have her hold the pendulum over her pregnant abdomen. You observe and record the result. Test your own instinctive ability and that of your friends the same way—just for fun.

The accuracy is comparable to that of age progression in dreaming—a mother's subconscious mind going ahead in time during sleep while her conscious mind is at rest. She dreams she has had the baby and "sees" it is a boy or girl. The subconscious is not 100 per cent accurate but is far more accurate than the 50-50 guessing of the conscious mind. What is your score, your friends', your wife's?

To illustrate the current interest in instinct and animal brain function: As I was writing this chapter an advertisement appeared in a national magazine picturing a dolphin coming up out of a pool of water to speak into a microphone which was connected with an electronic computer designed to translate dolphinese automatically into English. The computer company was very serious. Inter-species communication is not only possible but is probable in the near future.

The era we are now living in may be recorded by the historians of tomorrow as the "space age." However, they will be referring not only to outer space but also to the increased utilization of that elusive animal portion of our brains that performs instinctively—inner space.

Your function as a parent and as a companion to your wife is intimately related to your recognition of these basic forms of interpersonal instinctual means of communication. Your inner peace of mind, your sincere deep thoughts of love and affection will be received telepathically by your wife and child.

The closer the emotional ties, the more perceptive the subconscious mind. This is the basic reason why you, as a lover and husband, make the ideal labor coach and companion. Your wife really feels close to you. Your calmness and confidence will be imparted to her and utilized efficiently to meet the stress of labor. There is no adequate substitute for the husband.

13

Obstacles to Overcome

Obstacle One: the medical profession

A STEADILY increasing minority of doctors is advocating and teaching natural childbirth and an active rather than passive role for the husband. However, there is still a majority against this concept, some individual members violently so. Why? Many reasons. I think the first and most important is that they have never truly tried it. This is obvious in some of the statements made by the most clamorous opponents. If the old adage "Don't knock it if you haven't tried it" were properly applied, there would be no further opposition.

Another excuse expressed is that doctors haven't time to teach it. This was refuted by statistical studies revealing the shortening of labor, the decreased number of doctors' examinations needed and so forth, when trained husbands are coaching.[1] To achieve this the doctor has devoted only two hours a month to group instruction.

One would think that if a woman expressed a desire to give birth to her offspring actively and unassisted and found the act such a happy, joyful experience that she would like to share it with her husband, the very least the medical profession could do would be

[1] "Father's Presence in Delivery Rooms," by Robert A. Bradley, M.D., *Psychosomatics*, Vol. III, No. 6, Nov.-Dec. 1962.

to cooperate with her. On the surface this seems a simple request. However, there are deep psychological factors involved. Many obstetricians are looked upon psychologically as frustrated mothers, men with hidden desires to give birth themselves. This is never more manifest than in the degree of violent opposition to the mere standby role a confident, trained natural childbirth mother and her ever-present coaching husband assign to an attending doctor at time of birth.

In our experience doctors are very much needed by about 3 per cent of our patients, to do necessary Caesarean sections. They are also needed by another 3 per cent who, for various reasons, require to be delivered or medicated in birth. Of the remaining 94 per cent, after careful prenatal training, the role of the doctor *at the moment of birth* is so insignificant as to be almost belittling. We take a lot of kidding from our patients regarding this. "What am I paying *you* for? *I* did all the work!"

But they are expressing pride in their own accomplishment and are really only kidding. They realize that the most important work of their doctor is the careful preparation for the moment of birth.

We advocates of natural childbirth point out that prenatal teaching of a patient and her husband how to work together to give spontaneous birth is the *primary duty* of a doctor. Most training centers teach budding doctors only the mechanics of abnormal obstetrics (6 per cent) and ignore the psychological management of normal obstetrics (94 per cent). Pregnant women should be looked upon not just as baby factories but in a total sense as complex human beings with a mind, a soul, and a body. Natural childbirth could properly if clumsily be called psychopneuma-somatic obstetrics—mind, soul, and body preparation.

Another obstacle to acceptance by the medical profession is that the method represents a taboo-breaking innovation. The history of medicine reveals a reluctance to change accepted established techniques. The old taboo that a husband does not belong at the scene of birth, the old taboo that there is a magical halo about the attending physician which would be diminished or destroyed by the presence of the participating husband, and the oldest of all taboos, generating from the mistranslation of Genesis[2] that a baby's birth should be attended with pain and sorrow —all of these taboos are torn asunder by modern concepts of natural childbirth. This is a mighty big pill for the medical profession to swallow quickly at one gulp. It takes time.

Remember the words of Max Planck. As a lay person don't try to educate established older physicians to your way of thinking even if you sincerely feel you're right and they are wrong. Rather, keep looking until you find an already educated one, usually a younger one.

Most doctors are egocentric. This is nearly a necessity in the practice of medicine for psychological reasons. You wouldn't want a fumbling, uncertain Caspar Milquetoast in charge of your health or life. Most doctors in established practice bitterly resent lay people teaching them another way of doing obstetrics. You are insulting them by implying that what they are doing and have been doing for years is wrong and your way is right.

A teenage mother, daughter of an established doctor, tells how she had to have her third child by natural childbirth (unmedicated, joyful, walking back from the delivery room going home in two hours, etc.) before her physician father changed his resentful attitude and grudgingly admitted maybe there was something to the method after all.

For you the proper approach is to patronize the doctor who thinks and acts in accordance with these principles. Don't accept a patient-hungry doctor who will "go along" with you, but keep looking until you find one who shares your interest, one who will teach and encourage you. I recall one couple who had visited, and hurriedly left, seventeen doctors before they found what they wanted. I can think of no greater stimulus to a doctor to investigate natural childbirth than to have his office door shut with

[2] Helen Wessel, *Natural Childbirth and the Christian Family*, Harper & Row.

great vigor several times by hurriedly departing patients.

Today many magazine articles are written on the dangers of giving anesthetics to mothers, the ill effects of medication for the newborn, and on the psychological and spiritual importance of prenatal education for both husband and wife. Often these articles also stress the need of special physical training to properly perform an athletic physical event like giving birth. Experienced parents write about the rich emotional rewards of conscious birth time and again in lay magazines.

With natural childbirth used and the husband present, the mother and father are two interested, analytical observers. Some doctors are uncomfortable under such observation. They don't like to be watched in their work. Such an attitude reflects a lack of self-confidence. Keep looking until you find a doctor who is self-confident and takes pride in being observed.

Obstacle two: your parents

For a woman there is probably nothing more irritating than to have suffered a long, gruesome labor, to have been sickened with anesthesia, to have felt she suffered the agony of the damned, to have been hospitalized for days even weeks, bringing a girl child into the world—then to have her daughter grow up, marry, get pregnant, and nonchalantly give birth without medication, walk back from the birth room, go home two hours later, and then add insult to injury by enthusiastically raving about how much fun it all was.

I had such a woman call me in fury one night. She claimed hysterically that I had turned her child against her! I ought to be ashamed!

I couldn't figure out what on earth she was talking about at first. The story finally came out. Her daughter had happily given birth by natural childbirth principles, left the hospital in two hours, and headed straight for her mother's house. When her mother answered the door the daughter shook her mother until her teeth rattled and verbally hurt her even worse. "I hate you, I hate you. All my life you held over me how you suffered having me. You lied, I just had a baby and it didn't hurt a bit!"

I became a wiser individual that night and from then on incorporated the admonition into our prenatal training—don't hold it against your mother because she had a terrible time bearing you; she isn't fibbing. Bear in mind it wasn't her fault. She didn't have the benefit in those days of careful mental and physical preparation for birth. She was not attended constantly by a trained love-motivated coach, her husband.

Fathers of our patients are also an obstacle occasionally. They subconsciously recall the indignity of their useless, separated, guilt-ridden role and unwittingly resent the useful participating role of modern husbands.

Such unconscious resentment can be alleviated in most parents by having them attend classes or read the same material with you. "It's so different now," I've heard from their lips so many times. Indeed, thank God, it is different now.

Obstacle three: your friends

"Dahling, you had natural childbirth? How vulgar!!" Women resent women. Men whose only contribution to their wives in labor was smoking cigarettes in the waiting room or drinking nervously at the local pub will try to cover their own inadequacies by cunningly attempting to ridicule your concepts. Don't get into any heated arguments; their rigid minds are frozen in self-defense. They are to be pitied, not argued with.

As I have often said the greatest handicap in practicing this type of obstetrics is the overenthusiasm of the patients and their husbands. They often tend to make a distinct nuisance of themselves.

One new obstetrical couple presented themselves in late pregnancy. I mistakenly thought this was their first visit to the doctor and began the conversation with a critical question to this effect.

The lady snapped at me defensively, "I've been going to another doctor regularly!" I looked bewildered and asked why they wanted to change so late in pregnancy.

She looked dejected and frustrated and rather pointedly explained, "Well, we bought a new house. Our next door neighbor turned out to be one of your natural childbirth mothers. She told me that if I didn't have enough respect for my own children to learn how to give birth to them she'd never speak to me again! We have to live next to her, so here I am! We like our new house." She and her husband became wonderful, cooperative patients but I had to start with an apology for the enthusiasm of their neighbors.

Obstacle four: hospital personnel

In a recent letter Martha Nell Sitton, wife of E. L. Sitton of Fort Worth, Texas, said:

Hospitals are distinctly unpleasant places to me in that they are too often operated by personnel who have no regard for human dignity; this at least has been my experience with hospitals; I sincerely hope that my own experiences have been exceptional, and that not all women are treated as I have been. Most registered cows receive more considerate treatment when they have calves than I received on the three occasions when I had babies in a hospital.

Hospitals are very good places to be, of course, when one is really sick. This is because they are geared to the needs of sick people. But a woman undergoing a normal delivery without fear is not sick, and is therefore somewhat out of place in the average hospital, unless she can adjust to the idea of being treated as if she were sick.

If you are in a hospital which is relatively unacquainted with natural childbirth the workers may be skeptical of you. It seems ridiculous but it's true. I have seen some attending nurses, even interns, and especially anesthetists who by their facial expressions and attitudes show they resent a mother giving birth without their medication. Don't worry about it; time will change this. Ignore them. Mind your own business so well that they can't help eventually admiring you.

Only a few hospitals benefit from nurses and attendants trained and experienced in natural childbirth. If you are a pioneer, take personal pride in it and don't resent an occasional slight.

As times continue to change, hospitals that keep a man and wife together in labor will be doing a booming business, and the ones which separate them will be losing business. This is becoming evident already.

Don't waste your time with the inexperienced and the prejudiced.

If you or your wife encounter obstacles that are bothersome, discuss them *only* with another couple who have been together in prepared births or with doctors or nurses who are not only trained this way but even in the face of opposition have the courage of their convictions and the intestinal fortitude to practice accordingly.

14

"What If My Wife Has a Miscarriage?"

THERE ARE MANY possible causes for early pregnancies ending in spontaneous miscarriages. By far the most frequent cause is the simple fact your wife was pregnant without a baby or with only parts of a baby being present. Now, don't immediately blame her. This could just as easily result from defective sperm as from defective eggs. Nor should she trade you in on another model, because even in the healthiest, most robust men there is a certain percentage of abnormal sperm present in the semen. This is a "normal abnormality" that occurs in all other animal species as well as human.

Our French poodle miscarried her first pregnancy, then proceeded to litter the place with seven healthy pups on her next pregnancy—same father too. On the farm horses, cows, pigs, and so forth, also have miscarriages. They pass empty amniotic sacs or sacs containing only fragments of fetal material instead of a complete fetus. It is true that there are some women who lose good babies, but this is very rare and when it happens your doctor will investigate for possible cause. Miscarriage occurs in about one in five or six pregnancies in humans. If you see a mother with five children, stop and ask her; she's probably had one or more early miscarriages. It is true that some women have twelve pregnancies and no miscarriages, but it seems to be on a purely chance basis; enough other woman have miscarriages to keep the percentage about constant when a large sample is studied.

It is hard to estimate the actual number, as many women have a late, crampy menstrual period and never recognize it as a miscarriage or bother to report it to a doctor. Most miscarriages occur around the second or third missed period time, some earlier, some later.

What should you make your wife do to prevent such a possibility from happening in your case? Nothing. There's nothing known that she does, or doesn't do, that will alter the incidence. Grandmother was put to bed—and had just as many miscarriages there as being up and around. Many a woman harbors a guilt complex because she attributes something she did just before she miscarried as causing it to happen. These "somethings" would cover three volumes—lifting, riding in a car, intercourse, travel, worry, fright, etc.—and have no known relationship to the miscarriage except sequence. What follows is not necessarily due to what preceded. Just because more gray-haired men have heart attacks than non-gray-haired men doesn't mean we can conclude that gray hair causes attacks.

Do not let your wife blame herself for something she did to cause a miscarriage. Remember our out-of-wedlock examples who try everything on earth short of internal manipulations to destroy the baby, but fail.

The other way around is applicable too. If your wife has a pregnancy with placenta and amniotic sac present but no fetus in the sac, she will have a miscarriage come hell or high water, no matter what she does. From the medical standpoint doctors treat all threatening miscarriages *as if* good babies were present, for the simple reason that until the amniotic sac comes out no one knows. The general rule is applicable: If a good baby is present, it will stay put and grow even with irregular bleeding and/or cramps. If a good baby isn't present, the wise uterus will empty itself and try again later.

Some uteri need a little help emptying themselves and your doctor may choose to do a D & C. This dilatation and curettage of the uterus consists in stretching or dilating the cervix to allow the entrance of a curette. This instrument is like a long iced tea spoon with sharp edges. It is used to scrape, cleanse, and remove the now useless material in the uterus. This cuts down on the loss of "wash water" (blood) the uterus would probably have used to cleanse itself of unwanted material. If a woman passes all the material and does not bleed to excess doing it, there is no need to do anything except get her pregnant again, and better luck next time. Luck or chance, not management, will determine whether a good sperm fertilizes a good egg.

15

"Daddy Helped Born Me"

WITH YESTERDAY's unprepared mothers and medicated methods of childbirth, husbands were mercifully excluded from the delivery room, and the idea of taking a picture of the mother and child at the moment of birth was even more unheard of and horrible to contemplate.

However, with today's prepared mothers and ever-present husbands the birth of a baby and the radiant joyful look on an unmedicated mother's face at the moment she first sees and holds her child are something to be remembered always, via photographs, rather than something to be forgotten, via anesthetics.

Accordingly, under two courageous administrators of Porter Memorial Hospital, now Olof T. Moline and earlier Harley E. Rice, husbands are not only allowed to be present but are permitted to bring cameras and record this important moment for inclusion in the baby book.

These most precious of pictures, as one couple referred to them, have come to be known as "daddy pictures" and are proudly placed on page one of the baby book.

Grateful husbands have given us copies, which have now accumulated into hundreds of prints. They are put on display at conventions and gather crowds of enthusiastic people who just can't get over how healthy and happy the mothers look and how pink and vigorous the yelling babies are at the moment of birth.

As an invited lecturer at banquets I have announced that the audience may now view pictures taken by husbands of their wives and babies at the moment of birth. It is amusing to see the reaction before viewing (Please, we have just eaten!) compared with the exclamations of wonder and amazement after viewing (How can she look that good!).

On a rainy day in Denver a little girl brought her toddler friends indoors to look at books. The favorite book she selected to show her playmates was her baby book. Its first pages contained the snapshots taken by her father of herself and her mother at the actual moment of birth, as well as other views which included her father, taken by attendants.

Her proud explanatory statement to her playmates as they viewed these pictures together, "Daddy helped born me," was overheard by her mother and related to us.

Childishly ungrammatical as it may be, I deem those four words most symbolic of all that this book and my life's work stands for. Consider the first word, "Daddy." Daddy felt her birth was such an important personal event that he was there to help her mother perform it. It was such a happy occasion to him that he felt it warranted his taking pictures to preserve the memory of it. These "daddy pictures" constituted something worthy to show to her friends on rainy days.

In the little girl's mind was a feeling of having been wanted by her father as well as her mother—a feeling of having by her very entrance into this world made *two* people very happy and proud.

Compare the feelings forever associated in her mind with the anniversary of this wonderful occasion, her *birth* day, with those associated by a child who inadvertently overheard her mother bitterly condemn her *delivery* day as a most horrible experience, "Never again. That d—— man can have the next one!"

What effect does all this have on the mind and soul of a child? Compare the paternal effect of the man who states he always gets drunk at the local bar while his wife is being delivered and the effect of the man who maintains to all who will listen that the most meaningful moment of his life was being present at the birth of his child. How much closer is the father-child relationship when he can truly say, "I was there when you were born—and I have pictures to prove it." It is heart-warming to find how many fathers carry copies of their pictures in their billfolds and how eagerly they display them.

Note the little girl's second word, "helped." Daddy wasn't an idle visitor or a mere curiosity seeker. The concept that husbands help, that childbirth is a shared experience, was recognized in that child's mind at such a tender age. What a wonderful mother she will grow up to be. I pray that the Good Lord will allow me to be around to share in the harvest of these childbirth methods.

This little girl and others like her won't mature to resent their own femininity and bitterly condemn the passive role of their husbands. Their philosophy will not be "If men had to bear children there wouldn't be any!" They won't grow up to represent "momism." Their obstetrician will have little to do. They'll be wonderful mothers.

The third word, "born," ungrammatical as it may be, denoted to that child that her mother *did* something to bring her into the world. The mother was not possessed of something evil from which she should be "delivered." She was possessed of something that was nice—me. She was pregnant, a state of "preparing to bring forth." God did not intend babies as an idle gift from a "delivery service" but as a rich reward for a mother's effort in bringing forth.

Even the child's fourth word, *me*, has significance. "Me" was the star of this show. All this fuss and bother was for *me*. *I* was the central figure for which all the preparation was made, whose arrival was such an important occasion that pictures were taken by my daddy to make a permanent record so that *my* birth will always be remembered.

The *Ich bin ich* awareness of personal identity is contained there.

At the present time there aren't many hospitals which allow husbands to bring cameras into delivery rooms. Only a few even allow husbands. However this number is steadily growing and is destined to continue to grow, for there is no legal reason why, in a free democracy, parents cannot be allowed to share childbirth if they wish. If you are not fortunate enough to live in Denver and husbands are excluded from birth rooms in your area, then get to work and change things. Such changes were brought about recently in California under the capable leadership of nine earnest doctors with the determined backing of the lay organization I.C.E.A. Write to I.C.E.A. for advice (International Childbirth Education Association, P.O. Box 5852, Milwaukee, Wisconsin 53220) and buy a copy of their booklet "Recommendation to the Hospital Advisory Board of the State of California Relative to Administrative Regulation and Husbands in the Delivery Room, January 8, 1964." It will help you in your campaign to change any restrictive rules against husbands as participating necessary members of a birth team. If there is no local chapter of I.C.E.A. in your community, form one. Don't ever underestimate what determined lay groups can accomplish.

After you have gained permission for husbands to be present with their wives in the delivery room of your local hospital, the next step is to let them bring their cameras. Let us supply you with some ammunition to convince your doctor and the hospital administrator that pictures are a good thing. The reasons are medical, physical, and spiritual.

1. "Daddy pictures" are of benefit to the husband-wife relationship. They are objective proof of true togetherness in parenthood. Birth is thereby illustrated as a shared experience.

Such pictures place the moment of birth on a similar level of familial importance with the marriage ceremony, wedding anniversaries, and annual anniversaries of this moment known as "birthdays." Aren't these all occasions to be preserved by picture taking? Why take birthday pictures on subsequent anniversaries but ignore the original and main event?

These pictures bind the marriage bonds tighter and make family life richer, more meaningful. In my observation the divorce rate is significantly low in couples who tenderly preserve via pictures the memory of the moment of the birth of their children.

2. The role of photographer adds purpose to the role of the husband. In family-centered childbirth the low incidence of postpartum psychoses (nervous breakdowns) of mothers is related to the *useful* rather than *useless* part played by the husband. Women subconsciously resent absent, passive husbands who take no active interest in the birth of their children. Dr. Carl L. Kline in a medical article[1] discussing the cause of postpartum psychoses states, "One of the most frequently expressed sources of resentment (of a wife toward her husband) is passivity on the part of the husband."

"Daddy pictures" are vivid proof of the husband's presence and his active interest. Many women have remarked how their husband's whole attitude toward being a father improved and in some instances changed completely after he was taught the importance of his active role in childbirth.

3. These pictures may be beneficial in the psychological and spiritual development of the child, as suggested in the first part of this chapter.

4. The pictures are valuable in prenatal education. They give reassurance to the inexperienced. Probably no aspect of prenatal preparation is as effective in dispelling fear and anxiety in the inexperienced couple as for them to study copies of pictures taken by other parents.

It appears obvious that our main reason for inviting the hus-

[1] *Amer. Jr. of Obst. & Gyn.*, 69:748-757, 1955.

band to share in the birth experience is simply that his wife will be so radiantly happy in her achievement that he shouldn't be left out.

And there is really no good reason why, if they wish, husbands shouldn't be allowed cameras. Cameras have been allowed now for eleven years at Porter Memorial Hospital, even flashbulb cameras, as there is a separate birth room for natural childbirth that does not contain gas machines. Don't abuse the privilege and come dragging along enormous amounts of photographic equipment, but use just a simple camera you hold in your hand.

No ill effect possibly attributable to these "daddy pictures" has ever occurred. "Infection—cameras are dirty," some opponents may claim. Yet our hospital has not had any higher infection rate. "The photographer will interfere with the function of the nurses." Instruct him to stay on his daddy stool (formerly the anesthetist's) at the head of the table until the birth has occurred, and then give him permission and directions where to stand to take pictures. All of this is dramatized and clearly outlined to the husband at the prenatal class on "Labor and Birth."

If a few "medical Daniels" hadn't dared to be different we would still be treating all diseases with leeches and bloodletting. Yet it takes courage indeed to stand with a new minority against an established majority. Permission for husbands and/or cameras in delivery rooms cannot be based upon a majority vote of the medical staff; the concepts are too new. The administrator has to follow his own convictions. Your doctor similarly will run up against a lot of doctor opposition. Some of this will be good-natured kidding, some will be vicious. He will need a deep conviction in his innermost soul that husband-shared unanesthetized child*birth* is the better way and he will need intestinal fortitude to persevere toward this goal against the many obstacles placed in his path. Is it worth all the trouble? Ask the parents who have experienced it, ask them!

After seventeen years and over seven thousand births without a single maternal mortality I am deeply and sincerely convinced that the constant presence of a loved and loving husband serves to foster a state of serenity in the mother's mind which is comparable to or a part of the religious serenity that has aided some mothers for centuries to follow their instinctive abilities calmly and give birth actively to their babies. Your presence as a trained and loving helper will foster that serenity in your wife as she becomes a mother.

Index

Abdomen, and breathing, 45-47
  bulging out, 46
  stretch marks, 122
Activities during pregnancy, 109, 129-130
Adductor muscles, 102-103
Admission form, 30, 151, 157, 160
Age, ideal physical, 93
  and older woman, 92, 93-94
Anesthetic, applied pressure as, 6
  fee for, 158
Animals, first-stage labor, 22-27
  four-legged, 95
  giving birth, 8, 9-10
Atmosphere, quiet, 4
Automobile trips and pregnancy, 113-114

Baby, after birth, 71-75
  appearance of newborn, 74-75
  and blood in cord, 6, 72
  born in car, 152
  and breast feeding, 174-177
  caring for, 165-166
  and circumcision, 159-160
  engaged in pelvis, 134
  and false labor, 145-146
  heartbeat of, 132-133
  holding, 73-74
  in hospital, 161-162
  lying on, 33, 37, 100-101
  and medication, 15-16
  and mother's fall, 109-110
  movements of, 101, 129

Baby (continued)
  need for mother, 162
  voice of mother, 177
Baby box, 41
  and ligaments, 95-96
  location of, 83-84
Babysitter, 111-112, 130, 147-148
Baby-spacing, 174
Back, bending 88-89, 94
  lying on, 37-38
  massaging, 3, 41, 106
  sleeping on, 100-101, 102
  strengthening muscles, 99
Backache, 157
  and sleeping, 100-101
Back rub, 3, 41, 106
Bathing, and pregnancy, 114
  postpartum, 164-165
Birth, in emergencies, 89-90, 152
  following, 71-78
  at home, 27-29
  moment of, 66-68
    and camera, 196-197
  and squatting, 89
Birth canal, 50, 53
"Birth climax," 67
Bladder, and pregnancy, 116
  problems of and natural childbirth, 62
Bleeding and labor, 156-157
Blood, and umbilical cord, 6, 72
Blood pressure, low, 123-125
Blood sugar, low, 122-125, 127
Books for parents, 168

203

Pain, "after pains," 166
 and hypnosis, 142
 and pushing, 64-66
 in side, 117
Panties, removing, 139-140, 165
Panting, 26
"Panty rash," 139
Parenthood, 168-171
Parents, opposition of, 189-190
Patients, nurses as, 15-17
Pendulum and baby's sex, 183-184
Penis and circumcision, 159-160
Petersen, Mr. and Mrs. Gary, 2-7
Pictures, "daddy," 196-201
Pillows, and delivery room table, 58
 and relaxation, 2, 4-5, 33-34
 for sleeping, 101
Placenta, blood in, 6, 72
 expelling, 6, 75-76
Planck, Max, 188; quoted, 19
*Pocket Book of Baby and Child Care,
 The,* 168
Porter Memorial Hospital, 1, 4, 6,
 196, 201
Position, contour chair, 35, 57, 87-88
 "froggy," 99
 running, 166
 for sleep, 33, 100-102
 squatting, 53, 56-58
Postpartum, 161-171
 psychosis, 200
Posture, 94
 and fallen womb, 139
 and housework, 82
Pregnancy, and baths, 114
 circulation changes in, 118-119
 constipation, 117
 diet during, 125-128
 first trimester, 116-128
 and glands, 118-119
 and hair, 118-119
 and intercourse, 114-115
 length of, 148-150
 "pleurisy," 133
 and pressure, 116-118
 second trimester, 128-130
 third trimester, 130-135
 and travel, 112-114
 woman during, 108-135
"Prep," before birth, 30

Pressure, preventing pain, 142
 and transition, 50
Primiparas, 1
Princess Grace of Monaco, 14
Prolapse of uterus, 91, 136
Protein nightcap, 125
Pryor, Karen, 170
Push, urge to, 5, 50-51
Pushing, 60-66
 and breathing, 58-66

Queasiness, 122-125
 and car travel, 114
Quiet, need for, 24
Quinn, John, 19

Recovery room, 78
Reflex, breast-uterine, 6
Relaxation, and concentration, 30,
 34, 38, 40-44
 and contractions, 2-3, 38-39
 and first-stage labor, 25-27
 and floating, 111
 at home during labor, 151-153
 and Kegel muscle, 61
 positions for, 33-35
 practicing, 40-43, 105-107
 and swimming instructor, 110-111
*Relaxation and Exercises for Natural
 Childbirth,* 83
Rest, postpartum, 162-164
 in third trimester, 131-132
Restraint during labor, 37-38, 60
Rice, Harley E., 196
Rocking, and breast feeding, 177
 pelvic, 166
 and real labor, 154
 in third trimester, 131-132
 when to do, 98-99
Rooming-in, 74, 161
Rules, psychological, 108-135
 training, 79-107

"Saddle" area, 41
Salk, Dr. L., 176
Salt retention, 119, 120
Second-stage labor, 5, 52-66
Serenity and religion, 181
Sex, determining before birth, 133
 and pendulum, 183-184